THE TROUBLE WITH TRAUMA

KERRY HOWARD

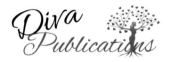
Diva Publications

First published in 2020 by Kerry Howard

© 2020 Kerry Howard

The moral rights of the author have been asserted

All rights reserved. Except as permitted under the *Australian Copyright Act 1968* (for example, a fair dealing for the purposes of study, research, criticism or review), no part of this book may be reproduced, stored in a retrieval system, communicated or transmitted in any form or by any means without prior written permission.

All inquiries should be made to the author.

A catalogue entry for this book is available from the National Library of Australia.

ISBN: 978-0-9954251-7-0

Printed in Australia by OMNE Publishing
Project management and text design by Michael Hanrahan Publishing
Cover design by Holly Fisher

The paper this book is printed on is certified as environmentally friendly.

CONTENTS

ACKNOWLEDGEMENTS

For My Clients – Every Single One of You

Without you, I would not have had the privilege of integrating my therapy work into the comprehensive trauma treatment that it is today. I'm just so grateful for the stories you have shared, the trust you have placed in me as your therapist and the joy of seeing you all recover and move forward with your lives. I am humbled every day to see the progress that you have all made. I thank you for sharing the laughter and the tears, but mostly the resilience and the strength to keep moving forward in your recovery.

For my staff and family – with this book you have all supported me through a lot of tough times, but you smile and chip in when I need your support. I couldn't do what I do without you and I appreciate the fact that you all go above and beyond.

Paras – for being a wonderful, open and caring person... My honorary 'Koumbara'! I will never forget your kindness and loving acceptance of my presence in your life. I really appreciate your generosity of time in being the first to review this manuscript and give me considered feedback.

Deb – for once again allowing me to share your amazing 'Beach House' to write this book, whilst relaxing on the Red Sea, snorkelling and soaking up the sun. I will need to find myself a 'retreat' closer to home until this pandemic settles down... But I look forward to the time when we can share a toast on your little beach once again.

Mum – for understanding why it's important for me to tell my story as I see it and that my perspective is not representative of yours about any event in my life.

From the bottom of my great big heart...

Thank you all!

PREFACE

In preparation for this book I completed a little exercise for myself where I asked myself a few questions about why I wanted to write this book, why it was so important, why it needed to be me, and why *now*!? In essence, my brain's response was, 'why not!'

Some of you may have seen Simon Sinek's work around finding your 'why'. Understanding that having a good sense of your purpose, your 'why', really helps to clarify a number of things in our lives.

In his book *Start With Why*, Simon refers to the fact that all inspiring leaders, regardless of their area of expertise, all think, act and communicate in the same way — which is the complete opposite of everyone else! In this book and in his subsequent books, he seeks to inspire readers to build a world in which trust and loyalty are the norm, rather than the exception.

In essence, when I go back to my 'why', I seek to inspire people to move from illness to wellness and even further onto awesomeness. I am a pioneer of radical recovery.

When I think about my 'why' — I recognise that what we are actually talking about is the need to have a clear sense of purpose for our lives. Having a clear sense of purpose is what helps people recover from the impact of trauma. We can overcome anything if we feel there is some purpose in our life.

My life's purpose is to help everyone to understand that what society thinks of as trauma isn't the reality of traumatic experience. As a clinician, I'm a trauma therapist and a proponent of the trauma model of psychopathology. This model conceptualises people as having understandable reactions to traumatic events, rather than suffering from mental illness.

Trauma models emphasise that traumatic experiences are more common, and more significant, in consideration of causation of mental health issues, than has often been accepted in modern approaches to psychological problems.

I have experienced trauma in my life; I even had PTSD at one point after being hit by a bus as a pedestrian. I could consider myself lucky to have survived, but rather I see that I made a choice to recover. I was able to recover with the help of a number of professionals, but also because of my own perspective about how our life experiences happen for a purpose; I just needed to understand what that purpose was.

The impact from any traumatic experience is directly related to our sense of responsibility in the experience, our lack of control or power in the face of the experience, and our ability to attribute meaning to why we had the experience. The key to recovery rests in our ability to feel a sense a purpose after the experience.

Trauma is normal — life is challenging — but truly empowered people seek truth, respect, integrity and purpose. Validation promotes action.

Sorry is NOT the acceptance of liability, it is the acknowledgement of another person's pain.

Resilience cannot be inherited; it is adaptive and imparted through a supportive environment where failure is applauded as providing another step in the cha-cha of life!

Human beings experience trauma because life throws us curve balls — we just need to learn to duck and weave. Dexterity is what helps us to learn. Without pressure, there can be no diamonds.

Show me someone who is truly inspirational and I'll show you someone who has experienced difficulty and learned from their experience.

Mental health awareness is at the highest level in humanity's history — but we are only now starting to understand how our mental health impacts all areas of our society. Are our mental health issues truly worse? Or are we just more courageous in our willingness to be open about our experiences?

Show me any 'problem' in society and I can link it to traumatic experience. Trauma isn't just 'mental' — it's physical. The sooner we call out Descartes on his 'detour' of the human experience, the sooner we may be able to turn humanity around to be able to make a revolutionary recovery.

Without storms and sun — there can be no life. Only sun — dry desert. Only storms — sludge and mud. No green — no growth. It is the combination that is powerful.

We can adapt to our environment; we can cope. But to be lush, we need a combination of both: sunshine, rain, sunshine, rain... Luscious! Without sun we have no hope; without rain we parch. We must have both and value both.

Revel in the storm, because when the rainbow appears the universe reminds us that there is hope. It's not surprising that the rainbow is the universal sign of diversity and hope. The pure joy of all of the colours in life, presented together, none more important than the other.

Our environment teaches us about nourishment. If unbalanced, we cannot provide ourselves the nourishment we need, and we won't grow even if we can survive.

Survival is Miraculous — Recovery is a Choice.

Don't be a passive survivor in your life, become a persistent recoverer. A revolutionary pioneer of your most luscious life.

INTRODUCTION

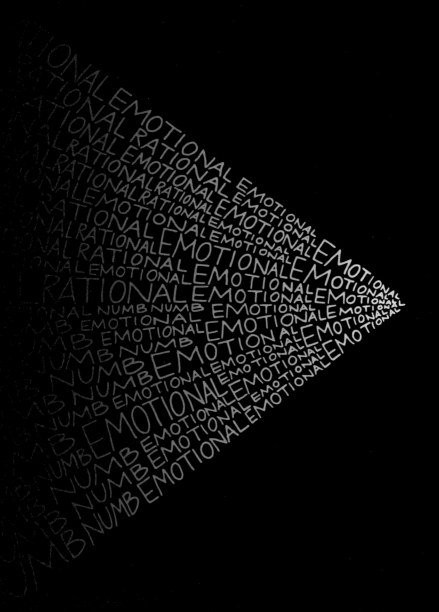

We Need Connection To Survive

Our ultimate need as human beings is for connection.

Why do I say it's our 'ultimate' need, a need that surpasses every other? Because without connections to other living beings, we would die. We are neurologically 'hard wired' for connection.

But what is connection? Connection is a relationship in which a person or being is linked to another living being.

CONNECTION AND VULNERABILITY

In Brené Brown's ground-breaking TED Talk on vulnerability (one of the top five TED Talks ever), which has been viewed over 35 million times on YouTube and led her to present a Netflix program titled 'Call to Courage', she talks about how shame affects our ability to form effective relationships — it impacts our ability to connect.

Brené calls herself a shame researcher and storyteller. Her research is based on years and years of qualitative research, interviews and observations that help people understand why the experience of shame leads us to feel that we want to isolate ourselves and protect our hearts from being hurt again. I deeply admire what she has done to raise awareness around how shame impacts us as human beings to the collective consciousness. (And I will always be grateful for the movement of TED for providing an innovative 'non-mainstream' platform that allowed Brené's ideas — and those of many other inspirational people — to be spread to hundreds of millions of people around the world.)

Brené's explanation of vulnerability, and how those who 'bounce back' from a sense of rejection manage to do it, has provided the world with a beacon of hope, support for being courageous, and an explanation of what it really means to be brave. She has inspired a new generation of people to develop resilience, and has done it by being willing to be vulnerable herself — despite the personal hardship this may bring her.

Brené talks about the challenges that we all face, and in this way, she really is able to normalise it — which is why it has been so powerful. However, Brené's research is only part of the story. It provides us with an explanation for what is happening and how some human beings appear to be able to harness their vulnerability, demonstrate bravery and act courageously. It helps us to know what behaviours lead to overcoming our human challenges, but it doesn't provide a clear plan for how to change our thoughts and feelings to enable us to act courageously.

We need more...

The need for connection is normal

Connection is an emotional need that affords us a range of physiological outcomes. We need to not only understand that it's normal and it has significant psychological impacts, but it also has physiological impacts.

As you read this book, you will understand how our need for connection is the absolute core requirement of our ability to develop as human beings, why we struggle without it, and what we need to do to change it. As human beings our whole lives are about connecting with others. From the time we are born, we are dependent upon being connected. It is the basis of our ability to sustain life. In our primal old brain, our amygdala senses that our ability to be connected is literally about life and death.

The difficulty with having our most basic emotional need being 'connection' is that our main problems as human beings then come from any form of disconnection, or a perceived threat of disconnection.

And this is the trouble with trauma: traumatic experience creates a disconnect.

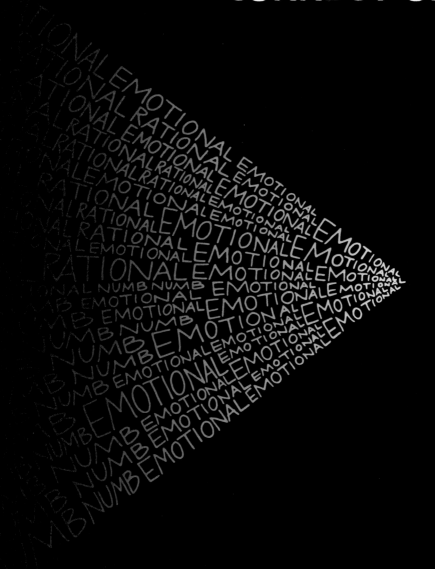

CHAPTER ONE

CONNECTION

If We Understood The Impact Of Trauma
And Taught How To Resolve It,
We Could Eliminate Mental Health Issues
In A Few Generations

As human beings we are neurologically driven to form connections, as being reliably connected to others is absolutely essential to our survival. As a result, anything that impedes our ability to connect is going to be problematic. The trouble with trauma is that it creates a disconnection. As human beings, we perceive events as traumatic because the event creates a disconnect.

WHAT IS 'TRAUMA' AND WHY IS TRAUMA SUCH A BIG PROBLEM FOR US?

Trauma is at the base of what psychologists refer to as psychopathology – the negative psychological problems we experience that cause us difficulties in life, the feelings and experiences we refer to as 'mental illness'.

It's important to be clear about what I mean by 'trauma', because many people, especially in western cultures, believe that traumatic events are only things that are life threatening. They think of events that are hugely impactful: accidents, rape, natural disasters. It is true, these events are absolutely traumatic... But so are the things that threaten our ability to connect, because to our brain they are *viewed as the same.*

The word 'trauma' comes from Greek – it literally means 'wound'. A deeply distressing or disturbing experience. Over time, it has grown to mean more, especially in psychological circles. However, I really want to come back to the 'original' meaning because I believe the way modern psychology has viewed trauma isn't helpful for understanding what it really is and how it impacts our development. My perspective is based on the original Greek meaning – it is an event that creates a wound, an emotional wound that develops from a distressing or disturbing experience. To our brain, a disconnection is a distressing experience.

It's important to ensure clarity on this point because when we consider the modern psychological interpretation of trauma, we have taken it to imply that an inability to cope with a traumatic experience is a failing on the part of the human who experiences it. Yet, the way our brain approaches traumatic experience is entirely normal — and arguably it is also completely developmentally appropriate!

We *all* experience trauma. Yet we are told as a society that we shouldn't focus on it. Our inability to 'not' focus on it, or to repress the impact of the trauma, is considered by the fathers of modern psychology as some sort of neurosis.

It isn't.

It is actually the failure to recognise the 'normality' of traumatic experience that has put us where we are now as a society — over-worked, overmedicated, avoidant, judgemental human beings.

We need to change this approach if we want to improve our lives, and the lives of generations to come.

It is the failure to recognise trauma as a normal experience that requires review and processing, and that is responsible for the majority of our mental health issues today.

I firmly believe that if we understood trauma and its impact and we were taught the processes to resolve it, we could eliminate the most common mental health issues from our society in a few generations.

How trauma results in mental health problems

My primary explanation for why trauma is so important to under-stand is that our very first experience of a trauma — the first that we actually recall and we can make an attribution and blame ourselves for — is usually from when we are about four years old. Our first experience of trauma is realistically earlier in our life, but the first abandonment we experience *and take responsibility for* is definitely before we start primary school.

Why do I say that this happens when we're four? Well, as human beings we have a really interesting developmental experience from the time we are born.

Needs

When we are born, our emotional needs are met by our primary caregivers, so our mother or other adults who looked after us as a baby. Our needs are usually always met; we are fed, clothed and have a roof over our head. In this way we can feel reasonably secure and can grow and feel nurtured.

Around 18 months old, things change and we find we start to learn language and express ourselves — we start to say 'no!' We are exploring language and what gets a reaction, and we see this as important, and we notice the reaction we get when we say 'no!', we will often repeat something to see the response we get. However, we do not have a direct or clear understanding at this point about what it all means — our little brain is trying to learn how the world works and we test certain behaviours to see the reaction. Do we get what we want or not? This will determine whether or not we should repeat a behaviour.

Desires

We grow a little more, and around the age of two we develop 'desire' — which is very different to 'need'. So, what's the big deal about desire?

As two year olds, we change our focus from what is given to us to meet our needs, and suddenly now have a *desire* for something different. However, we often don't have effective language skills to communicate our new desires. This is why two year olds throw tantrums, because instead of having a basic physiological need met, we want something different, but we can't communicate that desire to my parents or caregivers, or if we can they may not give us what we want.

The problem as children is that we don't understand why, because up until now they have given us what we *needed*, but they don't appear to do the same with what we *want*. We don't understand why there is a difference, because it's all in our heads and they seemed to understand us before. So, we think that our primary caregivers know exactly what we're thinking because for everything up until that point the caregiver intuitively 'knew' what we needed – we are egocentric.

But when 'need' changes to 'desire', we look to our parent to give us what we want and we don't necessarily get it!

Now, there are a range of reasons why we don't get it, but why do we throw tantrums? It's because we don't have the language to communicate our desires, and we're usually not getting what it is that we want, so in frustration we will throw a tantrum. Despite the fact that many psychologists believe our childhood traumatic experiences cause psychopathology, the responses we have at this age are actually developmentally appropriate. It isn't 'wrong' or 'bad' – it's *normal* for us to have this response at this age. If we didn't have this response, we would not be able to ensure we maintain the connection that is so vital to our survival as a human being.

From this point we develop more language, we become more aware, but we still believe that our parent can understand what's going on in our head. In fact, we believe that all the adults around us can read our minds.

Individuation

Then there is that moment when we know that children develop true and full individuation. Young children – toddlers – will usually be able to look in the mirror and say their name. I can point in the mirror and say 'Kerry' (in my case). I know that's the name we give that baby or that person I see in the mirror. However, I don't actually realise that the baby is *me*, that I am an individual, because at that point I still see myself as an extension of my parent... Until age four.

At around four, we work out that we can know things, or that little voice inside our head knows things our parents don't know unless we tell them. When we have reached that point of true individuation, that is the point when we actually know we are an individual and that what we think 'inside our head', our caregiver cannot know unless we express it. A four year old will come to you and say, 'I've got a secret!' This is when we become truly an individual, from this point on.

With individuation comes responsibility.

What I find quite amusing is that soon after individuation, we learn to tell lies.

Why is this important? Because from that point we understand that the things that happen to us happen because we impact them. What we know about children up until about the age of ten is they have what we refer to as 'concrete thinking'... Good things happen to us because we're good, and bad things because we're bad – simple as that, black and white.

If you reflect on your early childhood, you may be aware of when individuation happened for you, that moment around the age of four. You will have had a moment, after you recognised you were an individual, when you felt an abandonment or a disconnection from your primary caregivers. At this point, you rationalised to yourself that it was your fault.

The awareness of the impact of this moment is critically import-ant, because this is the child part that, later on, you tap back into when you are feeling rejected – your first experience of an abandonment. In fact, it is this part of yourself that forms the true basis of your personality or ego – the root of who you truly are as an individual.

But more on this later...

Shame and fear

We feel a lot of 'shame' from the experience of abandonment — remembering that at this time in our life we feel we are fully responsible for the things we experience — so we then spend our time trying to ensure we don't have this experience again. We are trying to avoid potential rejection in the future.

As children, when we experience that sense of abandonment our primary emotional response is shame. We decide we don't like how this feels. We don't want to feel that shame again, so we seek to avoid being rejected in the future, hopefully alleviating the experience of shame. As such, we start to become fearful about being rejected and we develop a level of anxiety, because anxiety is based in fear.

These are our two heaviest and most basic negative emotions: shame and fear. Shame is focused on the past, and later becomes the basis for potential depression. Fear, in contrast, is future focused and is the basis of anxiety.

This is a key understanding for humanity to recognise — all children experience anxiety, as fear is the most common emotion in our early childhood. So, most children of primary-school age experience anxiety. How they cope with managing their anxiety is directly dependent on their home environment, as the focus of security in our early life is directed towards our family connection.

In contrast, depression doesn't actually develop until later, in our adolescence. Interestingly, it's the primary driver of adolescence to work out who we are in comparison to our parents and family. In adolescence, we turn to our peers to obtain connection — we want to be like our friends, not our family. We are trying desperately to work out who we are as individuals in comparison to our friends. The inability to obtain a secure connection with our peers leads to increased anxiety, and ultimately depression. This is why the rates of depression in young people are recorded at around 50% — but

I would argue that *all* human beings experience low mood during their adolescence, we just don't all talk about it!

The impact of shame

When we understand the impact of shame and are aware of the paralysing impacts of fear, we can understand why Dr Brené Brown talks so passionately about vulnerability. You see, the experiences of shame and fear resulting in a disconnection can be moderated by the expression of vulnerability. When we are prepared to be courageous and share our experiences of shame with others, this affords us an opportunity to also form a new connection with another human being because we connect over our shared experiences.

The challenge for us as human beings is that our childhood experiences impact our capacity to be courageous. These childhood experiences have a psychological impact and change the wiring of our brains due to our human capacity for neuroplasticity — but these changes also impact our biology, our cellular functioning and our immune system.

Human needs

In 1943, a 35-year-old Professor of Psychology Abraham Harold Maslow proposed his theory of psychological health. He was the father of the psychological discipline known as 'Humanistic Psychology'.

In essence, this area of psychology proposes that every person has a strong desire to realise their full potential. This thinking reached its peak in the 1960s, and really emphasises the positive potential of human beings.[1] Maslow believed his work was essential to help us understand *all* human behaviour, and it provided an important contrast to the psychoanalytic work of Sigmund Freud.

Early psychological work had always focused on the mentally ill, but Maslow had a burning passion for trying to understand what made people mentally well.[2]

Maslow strongly believed that humans do not just react to their environment, rather he felt people were trying to accomplish something greater. Maslow studied mentally healthy individuals instead of people with serious psychological issues. He focused on 'self-actualising people'. Self-actualising people indicate a *coherent personality syndrome* and represent optimal psychological health and functioning.[3]

Maslow's hierarchy

In essence, Maslow claimed that our basic human needs are organised into a clear hierarchy, what he called a 'hierarchy of relative prepotency'.[4] Maslow's hierarchy is commonly depicted as a pyramid, a five-tier model of hierarchical needs, as shown below.

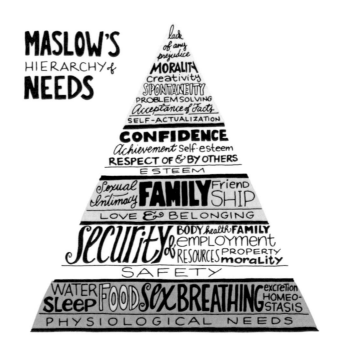

According to Maslow, the needs lower down in the hierarchy must be satisfied before individuals can attend to the needs higher up.

Maslow argued that the way in which essential needs are fulfilled is just as important as the needs themselves. Together, these define the human experience. To the extent a person finds cooperative social fulfillment of their needs, they can establish meaningful relationships with other people and the larger world. In other words, we establish meaningful connections to an external reality – an essential component of self-actualisation. In contrast, if our vital needs find selfish and competitive fulfillment, we are left with hostile emotions and limited external relationships – our awareness remains internal and limited.[4]

Interestingly, the way Maslow describes self-actualising people is very similar to what modern-day TED sensation Dr Brené Brown terms the 'wholehearted'. These people tend to focus on problems outside of themselves, they have a clear sense of what is true and what is false, they tend to be spontaneous and creative, and they don't get caught up in social conventions. They tend to be more open and willing to be vulnerable. Brené says the wholehearted engage in life with a sense of worthiness. They demonstrate courage and compassion and accept themselves for who they are and are willing to demonstrate vulnerability.[5]

In essence – they spend their lives being open to 'connection'.

A NEW APPROACH IS NEEDED

So, why have I given you a basic psychology lesson? I'm really just trying to give you the background to what modern psychological thinking has taught us about our basic human needs, and how the people who seem to be happy with their life – live it!

Obviously, if I thought that was the complete answer, you wouldn't be reading this book because I wouldn't have written it.

There are elements of this approach that are correct, but I think it doesn't quite explain everything.

I intend to outline why I believe Maslow's approach is in need of a review. In essence, Maslow's hierarchy is incorrect because it's missing the basic elements of the fact that our primary drive to have our needs met cannot be achieved without first establishing a connection. As a new baby, if we cannot establish a connection immediately, we will not survive because we will not have anyone to provide us with our most basic physiological needs.

Connection is our most basic need — without connection we are going to die. Any model of needs must reflect that without connection the rest of the needs are unable to be met. This means that our psychological needs are actually the most important for human survival... It is from here that everything else grows.

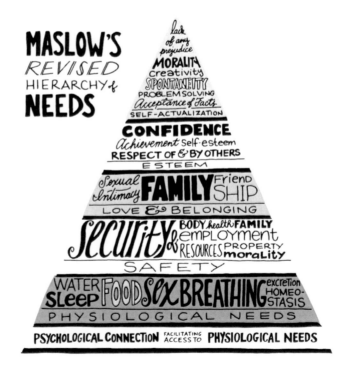

As I take you through this book you will begin to understand that the basis of every human experience is the ability to achieve connection. Our life experiences are driven by connection: positive experiences facilitate connection and negative experiences result in disconnection.

CHAPTER TWO
ATTACHMENT

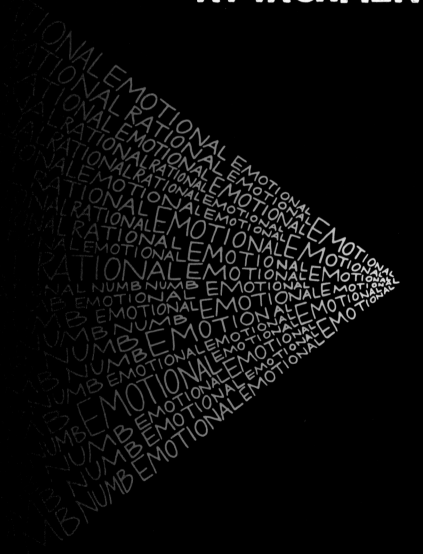

Traumatic Injuries Change The Way Our Cells Function

Anyone who has engaged in any form of psychological therapy, counselling or self-help reading will have heard about 'issues of attachment'. It's a term almost universally used to explain the difficulties we have in interpersonal relationships — the connections we form with family and friends.

There will be many who want to argue with my language, especially about whether or not what I am about to outline is really just an attachment issue. I sometimes feel we can spend far too much time splitting hairs and arguing about semantics, and it doesn't serve any purpose. In fact, by the time you have finished reading this book, I'm hopeful that you too will come to understand why the focus on the semantics — the judgement about what is 'right' or 'wrong' — is actually part of the problem!

I would ask that you allow me to take you on a journey... Try to allow the information I provide to sit with you, without judgement. Then approach this information with 'curious questioning' — questioning why you would argue against a particular point and starting to unpack the basis of your own belief system.

I want to share my journey of self-discovery with you and I hope that you find value in the sharing.

THE IMPACT OF CHILDHOOD EXPERIENCES

Developmentally, there are multiple points in our lives when the living and maturing organisms that are human beings, experience common milestones. We see this in many areas of child development, both physically and psychologically.

From the moment we are born we are driven by 'need' — we need to be fed and kept warm, Maslow's base of physiological needs. A baby cries to indicate they have a need that is not being met, and if they have their need met — they stop crying.

As a neonate, crying is our primary communication method; it is the only way we can communicate we have a physiological need.

This communication process facilitates a connection to our primary caregiver, usually the mother, that we have a need that is not being met. Depending on the quality of the connection, our needs will be understood and met quickly, or they will not be understood and will remain unmet.

This primary communication process forms the basis of our ability to grow into happy and healthy human beings. There is much research about how the quality of this connection affects our ability to form attachments, but there is not such a clear link made about the impact on the child physiologically in response to the quality of this attachment.

I believe the inability to form a good connection from childhood results in our needs not being understood and so they go unmet. The resulting unmet needs have a significant impact that changes our physical body at a cellular level.

There are many emerging areas of science which give us a good basis for such a position; from neuroplasticity to epigenetics, we are learning more and more each day about how the physical body is a constantly changing ecosystem. Like many other ecosystems, the individual human ecosystem can be impacted by factors that are external to it.

Our failure to recognise that we are a society of individual ecosystems which are mutually dependent, yet independent, is reflected in our lack of understanding about why connection is the fundamental basis of all human experience. As part of this complex system we have both external and internal experiences that impact us in a psychological way, and this results in changes to our physio-logical system. We are a holistic person and our system is fully connected − mind and body are one.

THE MIND–BODY CONNECTION

To understand why we have traditionally created a distinction between the 'physical' and the 'psychological', we must consider René Descartes and the Church.

Descartes was a 17th century French philosopher, mathematician and scientist. He studied many areas of these emerging fields over his life, but it's his theory on the dualism of mind and body that represents his signature doctrine, and it permeated his other theorising.[6]

According to Descartes, two substances are really distinct when each of them can exist apart from the other. Descartes believed that the body (an extended thing) and mind (an unextended, immaterial thing) were ontologically distinct. As such, he claimed that the human mind and body are distinct from one another.[7]

Unfortunately for the rest of humanity, much of our current medical and psychological beliefs are based on this 17th century distinction, as many of these early philosophical writings were the foundation for further explorations into anatomy and physiology – the basis of modern medicine. They also influenced the basis of modern psychological thinking about the distinction between body and mind.

Most of this early research and philosophical reasoning was also influenced by the Church. One of the only avenues of research into the anatomical makeup of the physical body was through dissecting them, and the Church was the sole source of human bodies in Europe during this time.

The Church had many concerns about people 'understanding' the human body – in particular the connection between the body and the soul. So, to be able to do any research on these bodies, there had to be a distinction made between the body and the soul. According to Dr Candace Pert, this separation has resulted in an 'unwritten rule' that specifies there is a distinct difference between things that are produced by the mind and what is produced in the body.[8] This 'rule' has permeated our society and become an entrenched part of our beliefs – yet it is completely incorrect.

Busting the myth

In her groundbreaking book *Molecules of Emotion: The science behind mind–body medicine*, Dr Candace Pert highlights that our mind is actually made up of a whole network of molecules that are connected right through our body — primarily centred in the upper body — from our torso up to our head. Pert outlines that information filters into the body from our five senses (sight, taste, sound, smell and touch) into our nervous system through a variety of points in our body known as the nodes of the central nervous system (CNS).[8]

Interestingly, these are the same areas that Ayurvedic medicine references as chakras, Chinese medicine calls meridians, and western medicine calls nodes — the core areas of the central nervous system where the nerve pathways from varying extremities converge and join together.

According to Pert, these nodes appear to be designed to enable ready access to the fast processing of incoming information to prioritise and bias it to cause unique neurophysiological changes in the body. In this way she outlines how our emotions and body sensations are intertwined in a unique bidirectional network in which each is able to alter the other. This process is usually unconscious, but may be raised into consciousness in response to certain triggers or even by intention.[8] The body can activate emotion as much as the expression of emotion can elicit physical responses in the body — they are completely interdependent.

What is more interesting from my perspective is that Pert goes on to highlight why the information processing that occurs at each of these nodes is impacted by our experiences, from childhood to present day. The brain records 'short-cuts' in the nodes of the CNS based on our experiences, and these are closely linked with the varying receptors associated with our five senses — some like vision are more complex than others, such as smell.[8] This explains why our olfactory system has a much stronger, and often unexpected, triggering effect on our memory than visual cues — as our visual processes involve more of the 'thinking' parts of our brain, which opens up the questioning of whether what we are seeing is real.

Pert references Dr Eric Kandel in relation to proving that the basis of our memory is actually a biochemical process that involves neuropeptides, receptors and molecular changes in our physical body. This work proves that our memories are not only stored in our brain, but they are part of an extensive psychosomatic network extending through our body, along the spinal cord, out to our organs and even to the surface of our skin. The intricacies of science provide evidence that encoding of some experiences only makes it to the nearest node before activating a memory and a corresponding physical response. This provides evidence for the notion that memory processes are emotion–driven and unconscious.[8]

Pert also clearly links how our physiological systems are involved in the processing of emotion and in particular how our memory networks are encoded, to save our brains time and unnecessary pain by ensuring that we avoid situations that would appear to be a threat to the effective ongoing management of our system.[8]

The body is a dynamic, complex system

Trauma changes the ways our cells function!

In another groundbreaking book Body Sense,[9] author and professor of psychology Alan Fogel explains that the body is a complex system that is 'dynamic' – meaning it is constantly changing in activity or progress and responding to its environment. He highlights that there is an interdependent linkage between our neural networks and our immune systems, also involving our hormones and our circulatory and digestive systems. These body systems are coregulating, and they are often all operating at the same time, managed by the various aspects of our central nervous system, but for most of us, in a way that we don't usually notice or pay attention to.

Fogel suggests that instead of thinking of the body as a structure of cells that form organs, it makes more sense to think of our bodies as a process. He goes into significant detail about the neurobiological reasons why this is true, and he specifically outlines the explanation for thinking about the body like this, as it assists in overlaying the scientific research that provides the evidence.

BODY SYSTEMS OVERLAP

CHAKRAS, MERIDIANS OF THE BODY & CENTRAL NERVOUS SYSTEM

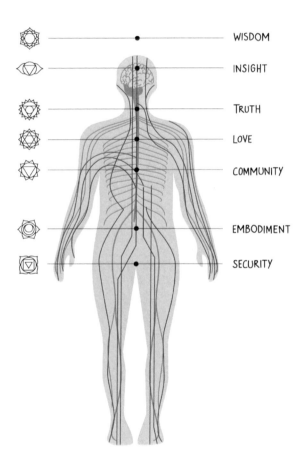

WISDOM

INSIGHT

TRUTH

LOVE

COMMUNITY

EMBODIMENT

SECURITY

The challenge is that most scientific research is completed in silos — looking at only one area of the brain or body and noticing responses that are localised. Worse, due to the nature of academic writing and scientific research, experiments are focused on the minutiae, rather than considering the whole picture.

Especially in neuroscience, the 'if this, then that' idea is extremely appealing. The ability to be able to clearly link something that is intangible to the physically tangible is something humans love, as it appeals to our concrete thinking, providing the brain with an easy and well-worn pathway to validate why something is happening that may otherwise not have an 'easy' explanation. In short, it provides us with an accepted link which quickly supports the acceptance that an issue 'just is' rather than being something that's within our control. However, even as science provides more fodder for the concreteness of our experiences, it has still been done in a way that doesn't draw all of the information together so we can see the whole picture.

If the information about the exact links between the neuro-scientific research and the physiological explanations is something you find fascinating, I would encourage you to read in more depth about this in Body Sense.[9] Just be aware that the information contained in this, and other books that I will reference, is often written for clinicians, health professionals and the more scientific minds. As such, they can often prove to be challenging reading for the layperson.

Rest assured, the scientific evidence for the connection between mind and body continues to grow. The recognition of our genetic inheritance influencing our biology and physiology is not refuted – the connection to our psychological functioning cannot be refuted either. As the field of epigenetics grows, we are able to see how our environment can impact the way our body responds and functions in an ever-changing world of cellular regeneration.

From my perspective, and the applicability to what I outline in this book, it is critical to understand that they are all essentially explaining the same anatomical areas within the body but in a different way. It is not about what is right or wrong, it is about acknowledging that varying philosophical approaches throughout history have actually all come to similar conclusions about the layout of the human body and what is impacting our system physically. This is extremely important to understand because it helps us to clearly see that the mind–body connection is very 'real' and not in any way discreet — as Descartes has made the world believe.

The sooner we can derail Descartes and his 'detour' of the human experience, the sooner we may be able to turn humanity around to make a revolutionary recovery.

It is essential that we completely bust this myth before we go any further, because it is the failure to recognise this fundamental truth about human life which has led to the problems we now face as humanity. It is the basis for all of our health problems — both physical and psychological — and I believe it is the basis for why our world has become a place many of us are not sure we really want to live in anymore.

THE FUTURE OF HUMANITY

We don't need to go far to find many and varied references to the 'problems' in the world — we used to have to turn on a television or radio to hear the news about how human beings are behaving badly towards one another, but these days the news is put in front of us wherever we are through our mobile devices, social media and internet connection.

There is a significant amount of psychological research which shows that people who don't watch the news are generally 'happier', and those who voraciously soak up all of the information in the news and perpetuate it are generally reported to be more critical, judgemental and generally negative. There is a link, but like most 'chicken or egg' arguments, it may be focusing on all the bad stuff in the world that makes people feel bad, or they could feel bad and that is why they seek out the news to validate why they feel bad.

In much the same way as I outlined earlier about how the ability to connect with others and share similar experiences can assist us to feel more positive about ourselves, when we see negative things this can validate our own feelings and experiences about our own negative life experiences. As human beings, we are always looking to our 'outer world' – our immediate environment – to help explain our 'inner world', the thoughts, feelings and behaviours we feel responsible for.

It really isn't surprising then that we have a new generation emerging who are using the 'megaphone' in their pocket to share their perspectives on the world. The constantly growing information superhighway that began to emerge from the internet and personal computing in the 1980s has resulted in our children gaining access to more and more information about anything their naturally curious minds turn their attention to.

We now have 16-year-old activists who were born into a world embedded in digital communication, who are able to share their perspective on issues such as climate change with the world – and they're heard. Moreover, they are able to engage vast numbers of people from varying cultures with a focus on the same issue – they have ready access to a natural 'tribe'. They are acting with passion, self-awareness, and enough ego to believe they have a right to speak up and be heard. They're courageous and they are comfortable utilising social media to express themselves.

Unprecedented opportunity

This level of public focus on our personal thoughts and personal lives is at a level which has never been seen before. It has resulted in a multitude of changes to the way we perceive ourselves and the world, and this has arguably been both good and bad. However, the willingness to openly share a personal perspective in a public forum has provided an unprecedented opportunity for humans to gain access to a variety of information sources and support to form their own opinions and share them – undiluted! As a result, such a young person can actively engage in debate with ageing world leaders who haven't yet worked out that their narcissism can no longer be hidden from public scrutiny.

The flipside of this is these young people are often really strongly negatively affected by the feedback they obtain through varying social media channels, as it provides them with a very 'live' perception of their acceptance by the world. As I am going to outline in this book, their experience of their external world is vastly different to that of their grandparents, and this has resulted in a significant shift in their self-awareness that has been both positive and negative.

We often hear stories of couples who choose not to have children because they are concerned about the legacy the next generation will inherit. Arguably, it is often those who are better educated who are making such decisions – so in the longer term what effect will that decision have on the overall collective consciousness? We are making significant decisions about the future based on our understanding of how our world is now – yet we know that the technology shift will result in things being as different in our world in five years' time as they were 30 years ago.

So, what should we do? The decisions of each individual do have a ripple effect on the rest of their community, culture and ultimately the dynamics and balance of the continued operation of the world. We could consider this in relation to Gaia Theory, the 1970s critically acclaimed hypothesis formulated by chemist James Lovelock, which proposed that living organisms interact with their inorganic surroundings on Earth to form a synergistic and self-regulating complex system that helps to maintain and perpetuate the conditions for life on the planet. Lovelock named the idea after Gaia, the primordial goddess who personified the Earth in Greek mythology.[10]

There are a number of movements that support the growing ideas within varying cultural groups about the need to change the way we approach our way of living; arguably the most universally accepted are the United Nations Global Goals for Sustainable Development.

In 2015, the leaders of all 193 member states of the UN adopted Agenda 2030, a universal agenda that contains the Global Goals for Sustainable Development. These are 17 goals for a better world by 2020; these goals include 169 targets and 230 indicators. These goals have the power to end poverty, fight inequality and stop climate change. Guided by the goals, it is now up to all of us — governments, businesses and the general public — to work together to build a better future for everyone.[11]

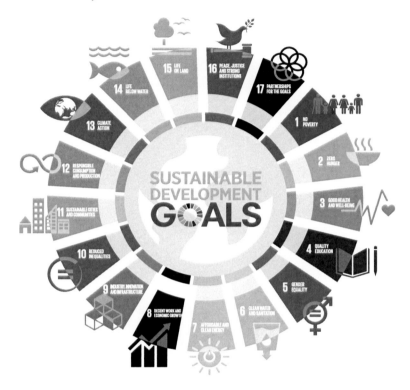

This aspirational set of goals may not have yet been achieved, but the key to achieving a desired outcome is about specifying the goals, committing to the goals and being accountable for our progress towards the goals. This book is written primarily in support of *Goal 3: Good Health and Well-Being: Ensure healthy lives and promote wellbeing for all, at all ages.* However, I believe that in implementing this approach we would have a positive impact on many of the other goals because we will become more aware of the impact we all have, both individually and collectively, for all humanity and our future life on Gaia.

CHAPTER THREE
VALIDITY

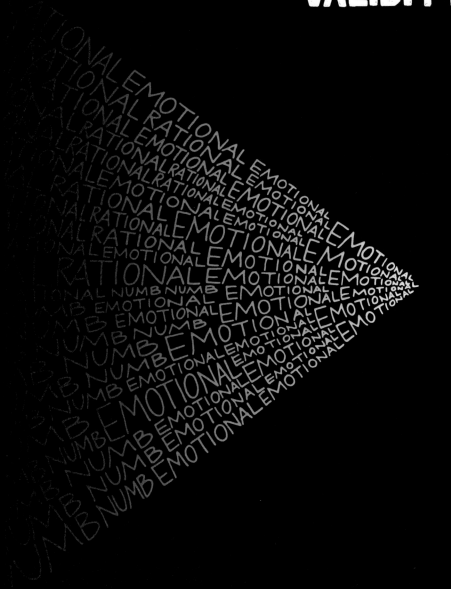

Humans Crave Connection
And We Fail Each Other
In Being Able To Provide It

There was a US documentary released in 2016 called *Resilience*. This research-based documentary highlights the fact that if we have a high number of 'adverse childhood experiences' (ACEs), in particular if you have more than four out of ten ACEs in your early childhood, then you are more than twice as likely to develop a chronic disease and your life expectancy can be reduced by up to 20 years.

This is critically important information for us to have when we are seeking to understand why there is often a gap in life expectancy between differing cultural groups.

Researchers in the US found that people who were getting ill at younger ages reported high levels of adverse childhood experiences. In my interpretation of their research, I'm saying high levels of trauma.

I believe there is a lot more work to be done to adapt the ACEs work to other cultures as a screening tool for the wider medical profession. However, what ACEs measures is traumatic experience, and when there are multiple events, it just highlights that the physical body is storing that information and is unable to process it, so it is changing the way our physical cells respond to varying life experiences.

HOW FEAR AND SHAME CHANGE OUR CELLULAR FUNCTIONING

When I first watched this documentary, it was like a light bulb went off in my head. In my clinical experience, working with many clients who had varying degrees of traumatic experience, I was aware there were often major health issues: cancers, immune diseases, inflammation and excess weight. I believe this is due to the trauma we experience in childhood and the negative environments we grow up in; these experiences create fear and shame, and that impairs our cellular functioning. Children in these home situations spend their time in early primary school years trying to 'control' their environment because they are justifiably fearful about what might happen in their future, and this can result in them becoming quite anxious.

The molecules of emotion

Many people are unaware that science has come a long way in the areas of biology, physics and genetics. It is possible to measure the vibration of emotion, and you won't really be surprised to learn that our two primary negative emotions, the two that colour our early childhood, are two of the heaviest vibrating emotions. They contract in their vibration. It's not hippy thinking — it's legitimate physics.

You know the feeling when you walk into a room and you think, 'You could cut the air with a knife! I wonder what's going on? Never mind — just get me out of here!' What you have experienced is the heaviness of the vibration of the energy in that room — the energy emitted by the people in it. If they've been arguing, it feels heavy and you don't want to be around it.

Alternatively, there are those other places where you walk in and the energy is really positive and light — you immediately think, 'This feels nice!' It's not just an 'ethereal' feeling — it's real. You can feel the vibration of the energy in the space.

For some reason, a lot of people struggle to accept that we can legitimately feel the vibration of emotion, or that vibrations exist in such a way as to affect us physically. Whether it's because it sounds like it comes from some 'alternative' universe, or for some other reason that limits our conscious ability to think for ourselves... I'm not sure. However, just like we accept that we breathe oxygen not because we can see it but because we know how it feels if we are deprived of it for any length of time, I would ask you to consider the times you experienced energy shifts based on your environment and the people around you for proof of this concept — just in case the science wasn't enough to persuade you.

This is a crucial element to everything else I am going to outline for you because it's fundamental to the way we need to approach our lives if we are going to improve things for ourselves, our children and humanity as a whole.

As human beings, we are living, breathing, moving energy. An ecosystem of cells that are bound together in a way that only some people can fully grasp – and I am still trying to grasp the concept! However, even though I don't fully understand it, the recognition that it is true has enabled me to do things I would never have thought possible in my conscious mind. However, one psychological phenomenon we do widely accept as true is that 95% of what happens and how we behave in this life is driven by our subconscious.

So, when we grow up as children in an environment that is constantly vibrating at a very low, contracted energy space that is created by fear and shame, it impacts the way our cells communicate.

CHILDREN AND ANXIETY

Unrelenting fear causes our bodies to vibrate at a very low level – constantly. If a child lives their early lives vacillating between fear and shame – the vibrational impact of their environment is having a negative impact on their cellular functioning. In my opinion, it's this effect that alters their cells and makes them more susceptible to chronic disease later in their lives.

As I said earlier, prior to the age of ten, developmentally we have what we call 'concrete thinking'. This means we believe good things happen to us because we're good, and bad things because we're bad. When we reflect on the feelings of abandonment that we experience, we feel shame and we don't like how it feels, so we seek to avoid it in the future – this is where anxiety begins.

Anxiety in a child can be managed reasonably well, depending upon what the family situation is like. Prior to hitting puberty, children look to their family connections to give them that sense of security and support. If they have a good, solid family base, even if they have experienced an abandonment, they can usually cope better than those children who have a volatile home environment.

As I have already noted, every single person on the planet actually has the experience of abandonment around the age of four; it results from some interaction between the child and their primary caregivers. For some people it's a huge thing, like getting lost or being involved in an accident. Yet for other people it's only a little thing, like being punished for something we didn't do or being put into 'time out' for too long or too often, but the shame is still enough to make that child fearful of a future rejection.

If the rest of the family situation is relatively secure, mum and dad are open and communicative and the household is quite stable, then that situation can work out reasonably well. From this supported space of security, this child can get through life without being terribly anxious during their early school years. However, if their home life is really unstable or volatile, those children are being set up for some major problems. As a society, we really need to understand that this is a community-based problem.

If we wait to intervene until a child is in their adolescence, we have left it later than it needs to be. We need to intervene with children when they are younger, in primary school, and start addressing high levels of fear when they are still young. We are aware that as children, our anxiety is usually triggered by something in our environment, but often we don't even know what it is that makes us feel scared and we are unable to communicate it.

This is really critical for our community. How many of us, or our family and friends, have been, or are, going through a divorce? It is essential to understand that if we have children in the divorcing household, even though it may look like they are coping okay, we need to spend time communicating with them that the relationship failure is not their fault. It is incredibly important to be honest and open in all communication with children about the relationship breakdown. Explaining to them that mummy and daddy still love them just as much as they did before, but they don't want to live in the same house together anymore. It is critical that these children understand that the relationship breakdown is not their fault and this needs to be reinforced at regular intervals for several years after divorce. Despite how they might appear, they are already going to feel abandoned and possibly rejected by either parent. I can't stress strongly enough how important it is to communicate openly about the causes for a relationship breakdown, without heavily apportioning blame.

ADOLESCENTS AND DEPRESSION

When we consider the impact of trauma moving into adolescence, the key is in understanding that as an adolescent, our job is to separate ourselves from our parents. At this point in our lives, we think our parents are the most uncool people on the planet! We really don't want to be anything like them — they embarrass us. This is perfectly normal. In our adolescence, our job is to differentiate ourselves from our parents and actually try to link ourselves very strongly to our peers.

Interestingly, adolescence is the first point in our lives when we are likely to experience depression. The focus on trying to connect with our peers is often the basis for why depressive symptoms are so high for adolescents. Clinically, it's quite unusual to have depressive symptoms in children, but there is a spike of depressive symptoms, or low mood, in adolescence.

So why do adolescents experience depression at such high rates? Research indicates that around 50% of adolescents experience depression at some point. I believe the rates of depression could actually be much higher, however the feelings of low mood can shift quite quickly in adolescence, so it only tends to come to the attention of parents or teachers when it becomes chronic.

You may recall that our first experience of trauma around the age of four results from a feeling of abandonment, a disconnection which is laden with shame. When we feel responsible for this disconnection, our emotional response is feeling shame for the perceived abandonment. As children, we take responsibility for this disconnection and we then fear rejection in the future. While we are connected to our parents we can more readily manage the fear. However, in adolescence, we don't want to be connected to our parents, we want to connect to our peers. If we feel rejected by our peers, the resulting traumatic impact is depression.

Depression is driven by shame, the heaviest emotion we experience as human beings, and we don't like how it feels. To try to prevent that feeling ever coming up again, our brain will often increase the negativity of the experience by constantly raising the prospect of 'if only' these things didn't happen. This constant negative mind chatter is called 'rumination', and many adolescents and adults find it very difficult to stop ruminating.

Now interestingly, this experience of feeling the shame and not ever wanting to feel it again is developmentally 'normal', and we have discussed that our first experience of this heavy emotion is around the age of four. However, in adolescence, when we feel rejected by our peers, we tend to become very negative in our internal thinking, and our very critical 'protector' part becomes much stronger. This is significant because these two parts of self – the 'child' and the 'protector' – are the basis of our emotional regulation system, but more about them later.

WHY ANXIETY CAUSES SO MANY PROBLEMS

In our society, there is often debate about what comes first: depression or anxiety?

As you can see, it is clearly anxiety that develops first. Our first cognitive emotional experience is shame, but the experience of shame actually leads us to a place in which we recognise that we don't want to experience shame again. Often the first significant experience of shame was quite a surprise to us, something that was completely outside of our control. So, we become fearful of experiencing it again in the future and we are anxious to avoid it, usually becoming as controlling as we can possibly be of our environment to minimise the fear of the potential shame. This results in a very low level of vibration, contracting vibrational space, that impacts the healthy development and replication of our cells.

When we hit our adolescence, we are trying to differentiate ourselves from our parents and connect with our peers. At one end of the spectrum we have young people who have a good relationship with parents, and they appear to be able to have good peer relationships as well – they appear to have it all worked out. We think of these people as the 'popular' kids that we went to school with, the ones that we wanted to be like and accepted by.

Interestingly – nothing is ever exactly as perfect as it seems...

If our connection to our parents is secure but we don't get a very good connection to our peers then it will have a negative impact. It may be manageable, but it still creates significant issues because developmentally we need to separate ourselves from our parents at this point – for the survival of the species, we need to find our likeminded peers who accept us. Young people in this situation are more likely to experience low mood that can become chronic, resulting in depression.

Then there are those who don't have a great connection with parents, not necessarily because they are openly abusive, but perhaps they are just busy working and unavailable. This is an upbringing I refer to as 'neglectful' – not because the parents are openly neglectful, but they often are not physically or emotionally available. Their attention is elsewhere. These young people tend to be quite self-reliant, and this can cause them to struggle with forming good peer relationships. They almost expect that no one is going to be very interested in them anyway, so they don't actively pursue connections with peers. Unfortunately, this is the norm of modern-day parenting, due to parents' focusing on career success and the focus they have on validating themselves 'externally'. This is probably the largest group, and these adolescents experience low mood continuously — but it's almost 'normal' for them.

At the very end of the spectrum, surprisingly we can find good peer connections. If we had a terrible parental relationship — perhaps it was abusive or your home life was very unstable — then sometimes we can get really good connections to peers. Often this happens because we connect with all the other kids who have big problems because their home life is also insecure and volatile. These adolescents often end up grouping together and re-bonding into a 'family' of other teenagers just like them. These kids will usually survive adolescence without appearing to be chronically depressed — it's interesting that juvenile delinquents can manage a little better by connecting with each other. They often manage better as a group, not necessarily getting depressed about it as such, until they find alcohol and other drugs to 'numb' themselves and their feelings of rejection... Then that's a whole different ball game.

Why is it that some adolescents will end up with depression? It's often because their family life has not given them the sense of security they needed, and they have not been able to get a good peer-to-peer social connection either. In this case, they often think quite negatively about themselves: 'I don't fit with the family, I don't fit with my peers or in the community'. As a result, they are more likely to become depressed.

THE DEVELOPMENT OF OUR NEGATIVE BELIEF SYSTEM

We establish our negative beliefs from childhood; in fact, our primary negative belief is 'I'm not good enough', and we develop this belief before the age of seven. Developmentally, this is also normal

– go back to our concrete thinking: black or white. If my parent or teacher is not happy with me, they are obviously cranky with me, so I'm feeling the shame of the disconnection and develop the feeling of not being good enough. So even if we had 'perfect' parents, we will most likely develop this belief in school.

Our education system compounds this by constantly comparing us to each other, and this affords us some awareness of an external hierarchy we have to compare ourselves to. This process is usually supported by our parents, as many parents will compare our achievements with our siblings or other family or friend's children. This is one of the major problems we create with modern parenting: we encourage our children to seek their validity *outside* of themselves, and we do it to them constantly.

So, when we hit adolescence, we really expand on our negative beliefs and they grow significantly – things like 'I'm different', 'I don't belong' and many of those self-deprecating thoughts and feelings. Why is that important? I have already highlighted how the focus really becomes negative and our 'protector' part of self gathers a lot of fuel to add to our negative feelings about ourselves during adolescence. In addition, we have a lot of synaptic changes that happen in our brains over this period, and then we throw hormones into the mix!

In my first book *Define Your Inner Diva*, I talk about life cycles, the seven-year cycles we have in our life that centre around our development of self. Our adolescence is our third development cycle (age 14 to 21), and it is governed by fire – it is very creative but there is also a lot of change – both psychologically and physiologically.

Each development cycle of seven years has a mid-point that also denotes a change point. Like most cycles, the first half involves a lot of growth and change, and the second half is often a reflection about those changes and a recognition that we're not 100% satisfied with what we experienced. So, in our adolescence we usually reach the second part of this development cycle (age 17 to 18) and we decide,

'I'm just going to be this "thing" [insert career choice here], and when I am this "thing" then everybody will think I'm amazing!'

This is often the path taken by the 'neglected, low mood' adolescents. In this way, we can feel more empowered to pull ourselves up by the bootstraps, coming out of that 'mediocre' adolescence, off the back of a reasonably disconnected family life in our early childhood, and we decide we are going to 'prove ourselves' by being great in a particular occupation.

The baggage

Often our feelings of being rejected by our family and being unable to connect with our peers mean we end up approaching life in one of two ways...

Firstly, we can feel we want to please the family so they will finally see how great we really are! In this way, we believe we will finally gain the acceptance and connection we have needed since childhood. We are seeking 'unconditional love' from them.

So, we go on and become whatever it is the family wants us to be, or something we think they will respect or admire. We feel a strong desire to be this perfect human being, to please Mum and Dad and *FINALLY* gain their acceptance. This is really about proving ourself and obtaining that sense of 'unconditional love'.

Alternatively, we might have decided we are never going to be accepted by our parents, that they will never love us unconditionally, and so we give up on ever pursuing our dreams. We have already accepted defeat because we have never actually achieved anything; we feel like a failure, and it doesn't matter what we do, it will never be good enough. We have already decided we will never receive 'unconditional love', so we start to reject others before they can also find us 'wanting'.

Depending on our circumstances, we may fit into different points along this continuum of how we approach our adult life.

This is important because when we get into a depressed space, depression is very much shame based. With anxiety, it is very much fear based. Depression is looking back over the events of our life, in our past. We look back and we think, 'If only this didn't happen, if only that didn't happen.' However, anxiety is looking to the future. We contemplate the future in fear, thinking, 'What if this happens, what if that happens!' There are very clear distinctions about what the difference between depression and anxiety actually is.

It is essential we understand the difference because in all the future connections we make, from friendships to intimate relationships and our family connections, it is our ability to make secure connections with other people that has a lot to do with how we experience life and how much of our time we spend feeling anxious or depressed.

What is important to understand is we *all* experience these feelings at different points in time due to the way our brains develop... It's NORMAL!

Growing up enmeshed or neglected

As I have outlined, our ability to connect has an awful lot to do with how we were raised. If we were raised in a family in which our connection to our parents was 'enmeshed', which means our life was driven by our parents and their expectations of us, we will grow into adulthood seeking approval from everyone. These adults experience anxiety — it is driven by fear of not being 'perfect' — an adult who lives life in a childlike existence.

Enmeshment happens in a lot of cultures, like European, Middle Eastern and Asian cultures, where the expectations placed on children by their parents are huge, but they are different.

European cultures have expectations of children sacrificing their own needs and desires to care for the adults — so the child is not expected to have a life outside of the family without the support and endorsement of the parents. In European cultures, there can also be a gender bias, so the expectation of girls to self-sacrifice is much stronger than for boys.

Asian cultures have strong obligations for children to make sure they get a really good outcome from their education, because the parents have invested a lot of time and energy into ensuring the child gets a good education and the child 'owes' them. There is a strong emphasis placed on education affording an improved status and income, and it becomes stronger in cultures that are emerging economically. However, these pressures place a large emotional responsibility onto the child. Children in these situations actually feel obligated to give the parents what they want, even if it makes the child miserable.

Middle Eastern cultures have strong religious overtones and obligations that define gendered positions in society. This hierarchy sets the tone for opportunities for these children in education and life, and they are given a status based on gender that establishes a strong power differential. By ensuring that the 'lower class' is not educated, these cultures are able to maintain a power imbalance that is never questioned.

These cultural obligations are problematic for a range of other reasons, but they are unfortunately very common.

Alternatively, for reasons other than culture, there can be lots of other emotional stuff going on in a family. If we grow up with a highly critical mother or father, and they make the child emotionally responsible for them, rather than the parent being emotionally responsible for the child — this creates big issues for these children.

In extreme cases, where a parent has borderline or narcissistic personality traits, these children experience a lot of emotional volatility and major confusion due to the erratic behaviour of the parent. Children learn what they live, so often the parent behaves this way due to their own unstable childhood, and as their child we can often feel that we behave in similar ways, which can create even more difficulties and hypersensitivity.

Even though these are examples of entrenched intergenerational issues, *it is possible to break the cycle!*

The opposite to growing up enmeshed is to grow up in 'neglect', which means our life was driven by us, alone. We will feel we were unimportant to one or both of our parents; we will grow into adulthood feeling strongly independent, but often driving ourself to do bigger and better things to 'prove' ourself. These adults can experience low mood but they're often very disconnected from it. There is a feeling that no one is ever really there for them and it is driven by the shame of not being 'important' — an adult who lives life believing that ultimately they will be rejected, by everyone.

In an extreme family environment this could be really severe neglect or abuse, but it can just be a case of feeling neglected in a family that was focused elsewhere. Think about a situation where you might be a member of a really big family and Mum and Dad were working or busy caring for others. In this situation, your presence in the household was just taken for granted — if you were around... Great! If you weren't — it didn't really matter that much. In these families, it was not like your presence or involvement in your parents' life seemed like it was really that important. For some people, this situation can feel like a total rejection, where they feel their parents wish they weren't around — like they are a hindrance.

All of us fit in that continuum somewhere — it's a bit like a bell curve. We have the really enmeshed ones at one end and the really neglected ones down the other, and then for 80% of us, we fit somewhere in between. Understanding our place in that bell curve is important, because whenever we enter into any relationship, be that with intimate partners, friends, work relationships or family connections, how we react or respond to any highly emotional interaction depends on our enmeshed or neglected upbringing.

CONFLICT IN ADULTHOOD

Any disagreement with another human being raises the potential for rejection. When we experience any form of conflict as an adult, we are drawing on the combined emotional experiences of our whole life in how we respond. Remembering that our primary emotional need is for connection, how we react in an argument is going to be determined by our parental relationships, and then this is mediated by how many times we have experienced rejection over the course of our life.

If in our adolescence we were able to have good peer connections then our reaction to any perception of rejection is likely to be minimal. These are often the kids who appear to be coping with high school, socially engaged, and regularly connecting with their peers socially – through sport and other activities. Those who may be perceived as 'popular', although they usually still have their own challenges with their self-worth.

Alternatively, if we've gone through adolescence and not been able to form good peer connections and we didn't have good family connections either, we would be more likely to develop depression. It may not be very noticeable to others, however it usually results in more withdrawal, and this then feeds our perceived experiences of rejection, resulting in a much stronger sense that we're really not valuable or 'worth it'.

Why is that important? It sets the foundations for how we behave whenever we perceive a rejection is going to happen between us and another human being.

Whenever we perceive a disconnection (or the potential for one), whenever we experience a trauma, we are going to react in one of two ways: child or protector – fearful and clingy or angry and rejecting. No matter which way we respond first, we actually will experience both sets of emotions – so we 'autopilot' to our base response and then we're going to flip.

If we grew up in a household where we were 'enmeshed', our first emotional reaction to any perceived withdrawal or rejection of the other person we are in 'relationship' with is actually going to be quite clingy and childlike. It often involves pleading and begging, and is grounded in fear, such as:

'Please, please don't leave me.
Is there anything I can do?'

'I'm sorry, I don't know what I've done
but just please let me fix it. I'll do whatever
you want to work it out!'

The basis of that relationship can be anything — friends, family, partners or employers.

On the other side is a sense of absolute protective rejection. If we grew up in a household where we were 'neglected', our first emotional reaction to any perceived withdrawal or rejection from the other person we are in a 'relationship' with is actually going to be quite self-protective, disconnected and strong. In this situation, our response can be more openly rejecting of the other person — get them before they get you:

'If you don't want to hang out with me... fine!'

'Back off — you're crowding me.'

'If you don't like it, don't let the door hit you
on the arse on your way out!'

Then all is quiet. It's crickets — right? Ghosted! All of a sudden — they've disappeared.

Sound familiar? Why is there distinction between the two?

Some of you will be thinking... I have done both! Most of us have – because we go first to our 'primary' reaction, and then we flip to the other when the primary approach still doesn't produce the result we are looking for – which is actually a reconnection.

INTERNALISERS AND EXTERNALISERS

Whether we grew up in an enmeshed or a neglected environment or some point in between, added to the categorisation of an enmeshed or neglected upbringing is whether we tend to be an 'externaliser' or an 'internaliser'. When things go wrong, do we externalise the blame onto everyone else, or do we internalise it onto ourself? This tends to be based on personality and attitude.

In psychological terms, we refer to the tendency to externalise or internalise as our 'locus of control'. This concept was developed by 1954 by Julian Rotter, and it essentially refers to the degree that people believe they control the outcomes in their lives (internalisers) as opposed to external forces beyond their control (externalisers).[12]

If a person has a strong internal locus of control then they believe things they experience in life are driven by their own actions – such as with exam results or whether they successfully apply for a new job. People with an internal locus of control tend to praise or blame themselves and their abilities. Alternatively, if a person has a strong external locus of control, they tend to praise or blame external factors – such as the teacher or the exam or the person doing the job interview.[13]

If we are the sort of person who is an externaliser, and we've grown up in an enmeshed environment from childhood, we're going to respond to a disconnection by reverting to child mode first – fearful of the abandonment: 'Please don't leave me, I'm really sorry. I'll do anything!' But then if that doesn't get us what we want, which is essentially a reconnection, we're going to do an absolute flip and start yelling and screaming: 'You're the worst in the world! I don't ever want to see you again. Get out of my life!'

That's what an externaliser does – that is throwing the feeling of rejection off the self and onto others, because an externaliser cannot cope with how it feels inside. Often externalisers have grown up in that enmeshed space, and when they feel they can't get what they want, they lose the plot. They end up feeling like they have to throw 'molotov cocktails' at everybody else because they can't cope with how it makes them feel inside, the shame that they feel from being abandoned.

On the opposite end of the scale, if we are more inclined to go into protector mode first then we are more likely to internalise. We tell the other person what they did wrong, but then push them away: 'Here is your "list of charges" – all the things you did wrong! See you later... Don't let the door hit you on the arse on the way out!' At that point, most internalisers are actually quite in control, but they usually use an issue as a catalyst. Once they have decided the other person is not going to give them what they want, and they believe that they will eventually reject them, they push first. Ghosted!

Internalisers decide that it's a done deal. They close the door and send people away – mainly because they don't believe the other person is actually willing to give them what they want. However, when the other person has actually gone, and they haven't come crawling back, begging and pleading, this is when the internaliser will flip into child mode. For an internaliser, child mode is withdrawn, alone and isolated – curled up in a foetal position in bed and not answering the phone. There's a strong sense of being rejected, despite usually being the one who did the 'rejecting' to feel more in control of being abandoned.

An externaliser goes into child mode first ('two-year-old tantrums') and then into protective mode ('screaming banshee').

An internaliser goes into protector mode first ('judge, jury and executioner') and then into child mode ('PJs and alone').

The clingy, enmeshed side is where that child part lives, so it's our inner child who's throwing the tantrum — it's our four-year-old self. We trigger into the part of us that first experienced abandonment at the hands of our parents and we felt responsible for the rejection.

The protector, neglected side is where our older teenage part lives. It is our inner protector that is feeling rejected already and decides to push first. We trigger into that part of us that developed to assist the neglected child to cope with the feelings of having to look after ourself. This part is usually an adult. It is the part of us that developed in response to the feelings of neglect and unimportance, and it's modelled on the adults we had around us in our childhood.

This diagram also shows our other 'coping' parts. Our numbing avoidant part, which is how we cope with things we can't change, but don't want to address for many and varied reasons. Our rational adult self, which is the one reading this book and thinking about our lives, what we want for ourselves and how to get it. More on this later...

WE ALL HAVE PARTS

Why is it important to understand that we all have both child and protector parts of self? Depending on our upbringing, we respond consistently and automatically as either protector or child, and then we flip into the other one. We need to understand that our protector part is the internalised protector of our inner child.

Our inner child is vulnerable and wants to be given unconditional love. I will let you in on a little secret — it is not possible in this world to receive unconditional love from anybody! The only living being that will give us unconditional love is a dog — and yourself.

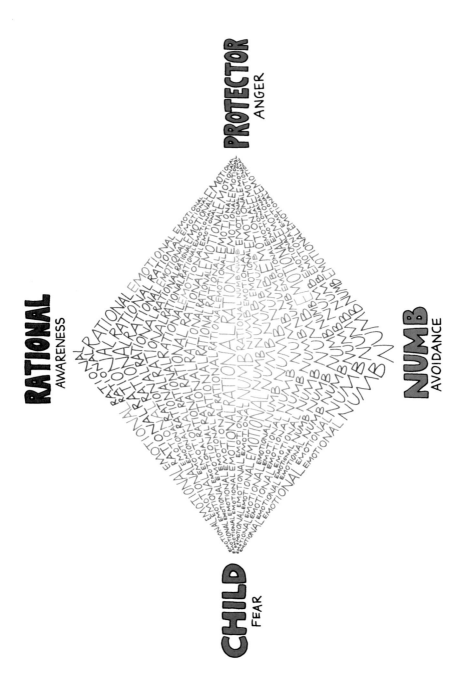

RATIONAL AWARENESS

PROTECTOR ANGER

NUMB AVOIDANCE

CHILD FEAR

As a parent, we might believe we love our child unconditionally... But it's not true! It is actually impossible for humans to love unconditionally. We love them an awful lot, and we accept a lot of things from them; we can love them fully but we don't truly love them *unconditionally*. Yes, I know that's hard for you to hear, but it's essential to understand it is a part of being human — not a personal failing.

It is critical that we understand this; we crave connection as human beings, and we fail each other in being able to provide it... Even when we really want to!

In all of our relationships and our connections with other human beings, we have to understand ourselves and where we are coming from in that relationship.

If we are reacting to someone close to us in hurt or anger, we have usually perceived a potential rejection; we feel that we are going to be abandoned. Our clarity and understanding of ourselves and our own feelings is fundamentally important, because in any relationship we have, you have to understand yourself and how you react, so you can communicate to the other person why you reacted the way you have.

When we understand ourselves, we can own our feelings and manage our behaviour better, through more effective and honest communication about our needs.

In my own life, I know I'm a protector first — I call her my 'Xena Warrior Princess', and she is very good at protecting my feelings by pushing people away before they can reject me. I disconnect from people 'after' I have read them my list of charges against them. What I want is for them to explain their behaviour and help me to find a way to rationally work through the problem. However, if I don't get something that is satisfactory, or it is just the same justification for the same unacceptable behaviour — I would just walk away.

Over the course of my life I became more adept at this, and I reached a point where I wouldn't really give significant others much opportunity to explain themselves. I observed a familiar pattern and I would walk away from it, rather than work through it to see if it was really the same issue. When I was younger, I expected that they would eventually come running after me, begging me to let them fix the problem — this was reinforced in my marriage due to the co-dependent nature of it. As I matured, I became more observant and I didn't give them much of a chance to explain or try to resolve the issues. As it happened more over the course of my life, my tendency was to cut and run, as I had decided the other person would never give me what I truly wanted — which is unconditional love.

So, once I push a person away, I really want them to 'fight' for the connection. I want them to show me their inner child and tell me how much they really value me and how they want to make it better — they want to resolve the disconnection. However, if they also have their 'protector' mode activated, they are looking for me to show them my inner child. But if I am an internaliser, I am not going to chase them, I am going to withdraw into myself and avoid any connection. I won't want to give them any opportunity to hurt me further by reinforcing the rejection. This will bring my 'child' to the surface, and I might find myself curled up in bed in a foetal position wanting to pull the doona over my head because I'm responsible for being rejected. This is your four-year-old self, and this part of you is the 'ultimate' controller of your system.

Yes — as human beings, our true leader is a four year old!

Something interesting happens at this point because my inner child is feeling vulnerable and rejected and then becomes angry at my protector (Xena) part and throws a tantrum. Think about how your critical internal voices work. In essence, the child blames the protector for always making everybody go away and leave them — abandoning them. The child believes that nobody is ever going to love them because Xena is such a horrible, angry, nasty person who makes everyone reject them. The child hates the protector for being such a b#@$h that no one ever wants to stay around.

Interestingly, the protector is the really critical voice. Our protector part is usually berating the child for being so pathetic that they can't be alone. Our protector has developed in childhood to ensure that we are self-correcting our actions and behaviours, to ensure we don't feel rejected again. However, because of where we are 'developmentally' when this happens, before the age of seven, the protector part only knows one way to manage the system — punishment!

In other books or articles, you may have heard the idea about the 'internalised parent'. Our protector part is modelled from our parents and other adults, like teachers or grandparents, from our early childhood. However, the protector develops a whole dialogue of its own as we progress through adolescence. By the time we reach adulthood, it is a strongly entrenched part of our system that feels completely 'normal', but it is the source of all the arguments we have in our head. Over time, the protector believes it is our 'true' self and wishes the stupid, annoying, weak child would disappear. You know what I mean because it is the part of you that gets angry with yourself when you do things that make you vulnerable or expose you to criticism. Many people will talk about how they 'hate' themselves at times.

This relationship that develops between these two parts of self is usually so combative that we just embrace this as 'normal'. The battle is not always raging, but the internal fighting starts as soon as we experience *any* feeling of rejection. Whether that is because our boss spoke to us about something we forgot to do, or didn't do well; or because we noticed on Facebook a few of our friends got together for a drink and didn't tell us about it. Whenever we have our rejection threat activated, our protector comes to the fore and starts telling us all the reasons our boss thinks we're useless; or why our friends really hate us and we can see how much fun they had without us.

In our society we have a number of names for this process. I am certainly not the first to recognise that it happens... But very few people understand that it is developmentally 'normal', and if we just had followed a corrective process, that we all regularly went through over the course of our lives, we wouldn't have to experience these feelings.

RESOLUTION OF THE SYSTEM

Our protector doesn't want to hear this because the protector feels they are the stronger part of the system and they just want the child to sit down, shut up, or get out of the system. However, the child is the actual 'leader' of your system.

I can hear our protectors all screaming abuse at me now!

This is the key to resolving the internal conflict. You see, ultimately the protector is actually the protector of the child! They coexist in a symbiotic relationship, but they have forgotten how they came to be. Recall that the protector develops in our own psyche in early childhood to help protect you from the feelings of abandonment and rejection you feel, but can't control. The protector seeks to give us some feelings of control over the situation, but does it in the only way it knows how — by becoming very critical of the child's need for connection and berating them for doing things that will get the child rejected.

As human beings we are all seeking unconditional love, and we do everything in our power to try to obtain it. It's this unrelenting pursuit that the protector perceives as weakness as it makes us vulnerable. That leaves us open to being hurt, and the protector's job is to stop us being hurt. Due to the point in time when we developed this part of self, it is built-in thinking — black or white; command and control. There is no grey area for our protector part.

Over the course of our life, our protector actually develops two sides: one that protects the child from external threats and one that focuses internally. It is the internal protector that creates the biggest problem for mastery of our system. Due to the point in time that this part developed, it is stuck in concrete thinking and uses force to motivate and change behaviour. As we age, the rest of our system develops greater self-awareness and is open to new experiences. However, our protector never grows up. They are stuck in our head, like the schoolyard bully who just screamed stupid taunts and called us names that didn't make sense. You know, the one that our mum would say, 'Just ignore them' — but we would get so upset! What's worse is that our protector forgot what their actual job is... To protect the child!

In order to resolve the system, we have to get the protector to recognise that their approach is not effective; in fact, it is very damaging to the system. We have to show the protector a mirror and help them understand 'who' they really are in the system and what their role is as an *adult*! There is a way I do this with clients that is very effective, and I have developed a guided meditation to assist you to do this work for yourself. I provide you a link to this in the 'Next Steps' at the end of this book.

So, we know our ultimate need is for connection and we want somebody to love us unconditionally... This is the basis of our emotional need as human beings. This is where it becomes problematic, because no matter what we do, or who we are, we need to recognise we are never going to get unconditional love — not truly.

INTERNAL SYSTEM

It's quite important to understand that as human beings we are actually a system of 'parts'. I have outlined our child and protector parts, but there are many other aspects to our system. Most of us are aware that we behave slightly differently in different situations — we are aware of the behaviour and in control of our actions (mostly!), but we can see the way we portray ourself is slightly different in different situations.

When we were young, we used to talk about our 'telephone voice' — essentially that is a part of self that is our professional person who wants to be taken seriously; we all have one of these. In addition, we may recognise some others. When we are in pain, our persona is usually more childlike, and our voice might become more whiney. We get the concept — we behave differently in different situations, and we can usually hear the difference in our voice, but we often don't even think about the differences.

This concept is really important to recognise because ultimately if you can master control over your own system, you can manage any issue that is affecting your emotions and you can learn a way to effectively ensure your system works like a well-trained 'team'. Like any team, you need a leader... We find ourselves in difficulty when there is no clarity about the leadership and a feeling that our system is just a group of disenfranchised sociopaths who are looking out for their own interests.

This concept is actually the key to being able to live a happy and healthy life, with full internal cohesiveness, valued, supported and free from negativity.

In fact, when we have resolved the impact of trauma in our life and you have developed mastery over your system — our head becomes very quiet!

It's weird, but there is no internal negativity or harsh judgement, and there is no need for second-guessing ourself because the part that is right for the job is the part that is in consciousness when we need it to be. There is cohesiveness between our aspects of self and a recognition of the value each part brings to the system.

Understanding our internal system is the key to ongoing management of our emotional challenges into the future — this is what I call your 'self-management system'.

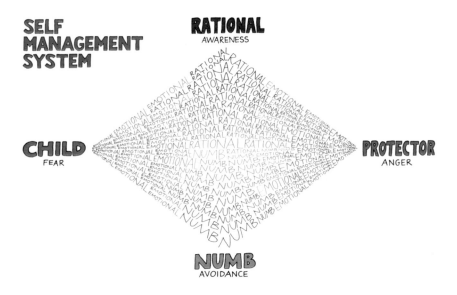

SELF MANAGEMENT SYSTEM

RATIONAL
AWARENESS

CHILD
FEAR

PROTECTOR
ANGER

NUMB
AVOIDANCE

Disconnection from our bodies

I mentioned briefly the feeling we get from the shame of a disconnection and why we try to avoid it. I talked about the 'old brain' and the fact that our amygdala is part of the reason this process is developmentally 'normal'.

When we think about how the physical life form is going to survive, we need to recognise that the human system is programmed to protect itself — to preserve life. The focus on the negative is entirely appropriate given the responsibility our brain has for keeping us alive.

There is a lot of information in popular culture about how our 'old brain' or the mammalian brain can cause us 'problems'. I think it's helpful to understand that rather than seeing it as the cause of a range of modern-day problems, if we could understand that it is biologically essential for our survival, we might learn to be more accepting.

There are a lot of 'positive psychology' focused people in the world who tell us we just need to 'focus on the positive' and then the negative won't affect us. No offence to that school of thought, but a big part of the reason this becomes quite challenging to do is because it is overlaying a shaky emotional system with a false outer coating – and it doesn't work in the long term.

We all know those people who talk themselves up a lot, make out to other people that they are perfect and their lives are awesome. They talk about everything positively, and tell those who share any negative feelings they just need to 'think positive'. But it's really very difficult to 'fake it until you make it', and actually that saying is a very typical example of how we, as a society, have encouraged our children and each other to ignore the feelings we have.

It's the tendency to pretend everything is okay that is a big part of the problem, and we actually teach our children to do this from a very young age. In western societies, it happens almost from the time we are born.

We raise our children to 'disconnect' from their own bodies. From the very earliest experiences where we take our babies into clinics and use 'controlled crying' techniques to try to get our babies to behave in ways that are more socially acceptable, we train them to behaviourally respond to our requirements instead of trying to understand what is actually going on for them inside their tiny bodies.

Motherhood is far from easy, and we are not given a manual for how to manage our newborn, let alone having some sort of inbuilt system for being able to intuitively know what the problem is. As our society has developed more technology, our disconnection from our emotional needs has become stronger. Not surprisingly, the mental health problems in society appear to have become more prevalent along the way.

There are several challenges that motherhood brings with it, both for the mother and for the child. Firstly, no one tells us anything about what pregnancy is like until we're pregnant — it's like some secret club we're not allowed to go into until we've paid our very expensive membership fee. And once we're in — there is no going back.

There are a number of things which impact the mother during pregnancy that also feed through into the developing foetus. It makes a lot more sense when we can accept that our bodies are made up of trillions of cells, and how these cells communicate with each other is impacted by a multitude of different elements. For the purposes of this section, let's just assume that our bodies are a micro–ecosystem. And like other systems it is in connection with, the growing foetus's system is directly impacted by the system in which it is housed while it's developing.

This shouldn't be that hard to understand when we think about what we know from a physiological perspective about things we should not do when we are pregnant.

We all know the things we do to our bodies that are not healthy, like smoking or drinking excess alcohol. These are things we know we should not do while we are pregnant because the impact on our body is such that the physical effects of these things are widely known to pass from the mother's body into the growing child's system. There is a lot of scientific evidence to these facts, not only about these known substances, but also about some other foods that can cause issues for a foetus — such as soft cheeses causing listeria. So, when we are pregnant, most mothers will limit the substances we put into our bodies, from chemical substances to foods.

We have even started to recognise this impact as a society, whether we have been pregnant or not. How many of you have seen a pregnant woman smoking or drinking and judged her harshly for her behaviour? This is because as a society we have all become more aware that what the mother is doing is hosting a living, growing human being inside her body, and what her body experiences is also experienced by the growing foetus.

The vibration of emotion

There is a significant amount of research about how we are able to measure the vibration of emotion. I spoke earlier about Dr Candace Pert's remarkable work around the biochemistry of emotion. Specifically, she highlights that the body is the unconscious mind and she confirms my position that trauma activates significant emotions that are overwhelming and that we store this information in our body – actually this is part of our muscle memory network.[8]

What isn't obvious in her book is that the biochemical processes involved in the expression of our emotions and the processing of those emotions actually cause our body to vibrate at varying frequencies and that these can be measured.

Quantum physics enables us to understand that human beings are electromagnetic (ELM) energy. We can measure our body's frequencies because our ELM energy vibrates or pulses. With every pulse, our ELM energy both broadcasts and attracts. Our energy field transmits our vibrations and magnetises other similar vibrations into our energy field. We are constantly broadcasting our own energy and attracting other energy.[14]

Emotions change our ELM energy and negative feelings pollute our body, making it feel heavy, whereas positive emotions are light and nurture our body. Emotions have unique vibrations varying from low and slow to high and fast.[14]

When we absorb a frequency into our energetic body over a long period of time, it permanently contributes its resonance to us. Do you recall how you could magnetise a pin or a screwdriver as a child? Certain kinds of tools and kitchen utensils are ferromagnetic. We can magnetise these and other ferromagnetic objects by exposing them to an existing magnetic field.

Just as we can magnetise an object, a constant intake of a certain frequency literally magnetises our body to that frequency.[14]

In essence, I spoke earlier about the fact that shame and fear are the two lowest vibrating emotions — in fact they are contracting. This isn't hippy science, there is quite a lot of research about the impact of emotional responses and how they emit a particular frequency and that these can be measured.

The image on the next page shows how this works.

As this image shows, the lowest vibrating emotion is shame, closely followed by guilt and apathy — both secondary emotions that are linked directly to the experience of shame. Then we have fear strongly in the centre of the 'suffering' emotions.

Our two primary negative emotions — shame and fear — are at the basis of our drivers in childhood. They are also the basis of our two major mental health issues in our adult life — depression and anxiety. Shame of our past and fear of our future.

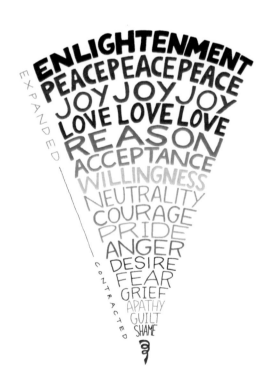

ADVERSE CHILDHOOD EXPERIENCES

I have talked briefly about the impact of strongly negative environments and the impact they have on our systems. When we look to the Adverse Childhood Experiences scale (ACEs), we see an assessment of criteria about the environment we grew up in and the impact of those experiences. The original research into ACEs was ground-breaking; they found if a person scored more than four out of the ten elements, those people are more than twice as likely to develop chronic disease, and their average life expectancy was 20 years less than those in our society who score less than four.

There have been a number of additional studies done since the ACEs was first published, and linkages have been made to criminality and mental and physical health issues.

What does this research tell us? That experiences in childhood influence the way our cellular systems develop. It has become so widely accepted that governments everywhere are scrambling to develop 'trauma informed' models of care for children who come into contact with children's services agencies, because if we can resolve the impact for these children, we save a lot of money in the healthcare system at the other end of their lives.

In Australia, the research outcomes from ACEs very clearly explain the difference in life expectancy rates between Indigenous and non-Indigenous Australians. That is not to say that non-Indigenous populations are not exposed to trauma, but the ratio is much more widely spread across non-Indigenous populations. If we were to consider the ACEs research, we could just as easily apply it to a socioeconomic model and find that the higher rates of traumatic events were experienced by people in lower socioeconomic groups.

If we actually break down the ACEs by the emotional responses, the majority of them are shame or fear based, with a bit of power-lessness and guilt thrown in for good measure. Some studies reduce the 'areas' of impact down to seven, but I think we can reduce it to two that impact our sense of security and safety:

Abuse: physical, emotional or sexual;
witnessed or experienced

Security: parent mental health and drug,
alcohol or criminal issues leading to volatility
and ultimately abandonment

There has been a significant amount of research into the fact that the ACEs is clearly linked to poor health outcomes, but not a lot of research has gone into why. Science is accepting that emotional volatility in childhood leads to significant physiological changes in the body of a child, so much so that they are more likely to develop heart disease or cancer and they have a significantly reduced life expectancy. We recognise that trauma is causing the problem, but do not understand the physiological changes that are driven by a volatile psychological environment.

The experience of an environment that is constantly vibrating in shame and fear is heavy, and it creates a lot of uncertainty. Think about our four-year-old self; the household is constantly vibrating in fear and in my individual thinking, responsible brain, I am blaming myself for the feeling of fear that I can't seem to get away from because I'm too small to look after myself. All children believe that adults are perfect — so they take responsibility for everything that goes wrong around them. I'm going to feel shame about the fact that somehow I must be responsible for this and am powerless to get out of it.

That environment leaves an imprint on my physiological system. In the same way we understand chemicals would impact a growing foetus, a strongly negative emotional environment impacts the cellular development of a young child. This impacts the child in ways that are very physiologically real, but the real cause of the alteration is not recognised by society at large because it's 'just a feeling'.

EXTERNALISATION

In fact, we are really good at training our children to deny the impact of their experiences. We have done this for generations, and it needs to stop.

I highlighted earlier how in western societies we teach our babies to disconnect from their physical needs by ignoring their psychologically driven behaviours. Controlled crying is one such technique we use to 'train' our babies. I think one of the most challenging things to hear is when people talk about a 'bad' baby or a 'difficult' baby. Babies are not driven by anything more than need – they have no concept of 'naughty', and when they communicate their need for connection in the only way they know how, by crying, we have an obligation to try to work out what is wrong and help them to resolve their discomfort.

There are many and varied stories of western parents who travel to orphanages in other countries such as China or the Ukraine. These are two of a few countries in the world that still have large institutional orphanages. Anyone who has tried to adopt a baby in western society finds that there are few options in countries where termination has been legalised. In addition, most of these countries have also decentralised children in government care and most of them go into foster care arrangements rather than large institutions.

These excited 'soon to be' adoptive western parents will comment about how placid and quiet the babies are, how 'well behaved' they are, that they just sit quietly in their cribs – not crying or demanding attention.

What they are witnessing is actually not a positive, they are observing babies who have given up crying or demanding attention because they have already learned that there is no point in crying as it doesn't elicit the expected response, e.g. they are picked up. Instead, they have learned that it doesn't matter how much we cry, we will be fed at certain times and our physical needs will be met at those times, but they learn to suppress their emotional needs as they have never been met.

It is quite common for parents of foreign adopted children to report that their new baby doesn't like to be held and doesn't cry much. As neonates, humans are incredibly adaptive and the primary role of our mind is to keep us alive. We only have one primary form of communication at this point in our lives and if we learn to suppress the natural response to need at this point in time, we become hard wired to it.

So, these babies adapt; they learn that there is no point in crying because it doesn't change anything. They stop crying because they know no one is listening. They don't fuss; they have learned that their natural instinct doesn't get them what they need, so their natural instinct gets extinguished. To a lesser extent, this is what we do in western society when we 'train' our babies to 'self-soothe'. We train an organism that is dependent to not be too demanding — what conditioning does that child receive? That they are unimportant!

THE PROBLEM WITH MODERN PARENTING

There are a number of reasons why modern parenting may actually be contributing to the increase in mental health issues. It's not about individual parenting techniques, but more about how the society, in its invalidation of motherhood, has actually created bigger issues.

We train our children from birth to not express their needs unnecessarily. Is it any wonder they grow up wondering if they will actually survive? Just because we are unable to understand the communication system the baby has is no reason to decide that their communication is inappropriate. They are crying out for a

connection, and when they don't get it, they experience a disconnect. Trauma. A disturbing event that leaves a wound.

As they grow up, we continue to teach them to dissociate from
their own body and their experiences. There are normal behavioural
training things we do as parents to ensure our children are kept safe,
but the way the child stores the belief about themselves in response
to this guidance varies greatly – depending on their home environment and the parenting style they receive. Consistency produces
security and volatility produces fear and shame.

Let's look at one of the simplest things we need to consider about
how a lack of time and attention can impact the way we invalidate
our children's experiences. I often find that analogies are helpful
when trying to explain challenges.

I want you to imagine you observe a mother and child. They
may be in a hurry to get somewhere, and the child trips and falls,
scraping her knee. What is the first thing our society does to 'validate'
if the scraped knee is a 'legitimate' issue? In many western societies
we have a cultural qualifier for whether or not a physical injury is
serious... It's the presence of blood.

The child might be crying and complaining about the pain of the
scrape, but if there is no blood, we tell her it's 'fine'! 'You're okay...
There's no blood!' It's as if the presence of blood defines the legiti-
macy of the experience of pain. 'Come on, you're fine... Let's go!'

Then we usually try to distract them by actively shifting
their focus onto something else, simultaneously encouraging their
denial of pain. Their knowledge at this point in their development
is completely dependent on us as care giver; if we invalidate their
experience, their brain doesn't counter that well. We actively teach
our children to dissociate from what they are experiencing within
their own body!

However, I want us to consider the alternative... Instead of
diverting the child from their experience and invalidating their
pain, what happens if we acknowledge it and give it focus. If we say,

'Oh, Darling... That must have hurt! Let me kiss it better!' Without exception, they would immediately feel better — whether there is blood or not!

However, in affording the child validation, we allow their brain to link to the fact that they have a legitimate physiological issue impacting their body.

Now, I can already hear the naysayers calling out the molly-coddling as creating children who are incapable of 'self-soothing'. I really want to scrub that phrase from the English language. As if, somehow just by acknowledging that a child has a physically painful experience, we are creating a person who is incapable of working their way through pain... Perhaps it would be better if we didn't train our children to dissociate from their pain.

It is important that we recognise we are not merely mollycoddling a child when we validate their pain; by attenuating their brain to the source of their pain, and affording their experience some validation, we allow a whole bunch of physiological things to happen at once. The acknowledgement not only provides an emotional validation and support of their experience, their brain needs us to affirm their experience is real so their own physiological activation kicks in to release a bunch of numbing neurotransmitters at the source of their pain. This also facilitates in the immune system the activation that allows the healing cells to kick in.

You can imagine what happens at the next level of impact, when I'm being physically hurt by the person who validates all of my thinking in relation to my physical body. My brain cannot reconcile the experience, and stronger dissociative abilities are developed. We know early experiences of abuse are more likely to result in increased levels of dissociation — it's conditioning.

There are multiple factors involved in developing very strong ties to external validation of our experiences, and a lot of them are cultural.

None of us are perfect parents; we all make mistakes. I say to any of my clients who are parents that we just need to accept we are going to screw our children up! Most of us are not trying to screw them up, but the reality is the way we behave towards our children is only half the story. Our motivation behind our behaviour is usually completely different to how our children perceive it. This is the joy of individuality, but it is strongly influenced by parenting style. Unfortunately for us as parents, no matter how positive our intentions, we have little control over how our child perceives our actions.

Developmentally, up until the age of about seven they are quite insular, and they don't make direct comparisons between themselves and others. From around four they take responsibility, but they don't make comparisons until later. This is one of the milestone points at which we should start to routinely 'normalise' negative experiences. The start of our psychological life 'spring cleaning' process. There are a number of areas of psychoeducation we now routinely teach children through school, but psychoeducation creates awareness; it doesn't afford a way to process any of the traumatic impacts on our physical system.

One of the ways that society has tried to combat the impact of ACEs is by training children in strengths-based psychological reinforcement. This is providing the child with validity of the fact that their environment is not right and should not be tolerated, which is better than nothing at all. However, I want you to think about the brain's natural tendency to focus on the negative, because biologically it's the negative that is the biggest threat to the living organism.

I'm not saying we shouldn't support the development of a strengths-based approach, but we have to recognise it is just 'one' tool children should be provided with to support them in their healthy development 'despite' their environment. However, I wonder if we would get further if we were able to 'normalise' parents to the fact that their behaviour towards their child is driven by their own traumatic experiences and there is a way the impact of trauma could be resolved? By highlighting the right and wrong around adult behaviour and educating children around strengths, encouraging them to speak up for themselves, we may be creating more psychological issues. We have to consider the impact of raising an expectation in the child that legitimises the fact that their home environment is unsafe and it's not right, yet we don't remove them from the threat. What message does that send?

It's important we try to take a broader approach, across the whole of society. It's not going to be a quick fix, but if we continue to pretend it will just fix itself, we will continue to spiral into self-destruction.

GATE CONTROL THEORY

One possible explanation for why the acknowledgement of pain might actually result in the reduction of the experience of pain is gate control theory. Originally developed by Melzack and Wall in 1965[15], they proposed that activating nerve fibres that do not transmit pain signals, called nonnociceptive fibres, can interfere with signals emitted from pain fibres, thereby inhibiting pain. The best example of this idea in action is when we rub the surface of the skin to offset the experience of pain, like when we have hit ourselves against something. Interestingly, this is a process that we do almost instinctively.

Recall earlier in this book where I referred to Dr Candace Pert's work on the molecular functioning of emotions — there is a lot of information coming out of neuroscience research to support the notion we need to afford the brain the validation of the experience of pain in order to assist the body to resolve the perception of it.

When we 'rub' an area that is painful we may be activating other nerves that confuse the CNS, but we are also 'validating' the experience of pain that we are having. As children, we need to be provided validation of our experiences from our parents, or other authority figure, to give rise to our brains connecting the messages received through a combination of senses. It therefore makes sense that if those messages are 'confused' in the input, that our brain is not able to provide the most comprehensive response to address the issue – neither physically nor psychologically.

Our children do not need to learn to 'self-soothe' – they need to have the reality of their experiences validated so that they can activate all of their available resources to correct the imbalance in their bodies as soon as possible. In this way we are teaching our children to be fully embodied – in touch with their bodies and in control of engaging in activities that help them to cope with anything that comes their way in full awareness – not by repressing their experiences.

Alan Fogel in his book *Body Sense,* talks about the fact that many societies often prefer suppression of expression in favour of allowing a child to express their feelings of pain or discomfort, that somehow it is perceived as the expression of maturity to be able to inhibit expression of things we find difficult.[9] Yet, it would appear that imposing this ability too early on a child sets up a pattern of behaviour that results in increased dissociation and disconnection from our physical body, and this lack of self-awareness is disastrous for the long-term physiological functioning of our bodies.

I'm not a neuroscientist, but I have read quite extensively about varying different elements of our biological make-up that could provide an explanation for how our body is providing physiological responses that can be measured. One such example is an enzyme known as COMT. Catechol-O-methyltransferase (COMT) is an enzyme that inactivates biologically-active catechols, including the important neurotransmitters dopamine, noradrenaline and adrenaline. These neurotransmitters are involved in numerous physiological processes, including modulation of pain.

Controversy exists about the pre-eminence and orientation of the membrane-bound COMT and its role in the CNS. It appears to play a more significant role in pain peripherally, so could be involved in our acknowledgement of pain when we 'kiss it better'. COMT is primarily produced in the liver and appears to have links to mental health, pain and reproductive systems. I am not sure about the actual involvement of COMT in the functioning of our emotion and pain systems; in fact, I think a lot of scientists are still trying to work it out. However, it is possible that it could explain a lot about the linkages between mental health, pain and reproductive functions.

I don't presume to have all the answers, and in many areas I find myself asking more questions about what might underpin these experiences. However, I know we need to change the way we think about the interactions between our mind and body if we have a hope of being able to resolve our modern health challenges.

It is through the miracle of neuroscience, of which we have really only begun to learn more in the past ten years or so, with the advancement in technology from fMRI scanning. With the development of our understanding of epigenetics and new insights into neurological processes, we are learning more and more that our physiological and psychological elements are clearly linked – they are not separate as Descartes has led modern medicine to believe. If we don't begin to change our perceptions of ourselves and our whole being, we will not be able to take action to allow our bodies and psyches to become one and heal ourselves.

The ability to change these things is only possible when we start validating our experiences, and this starts with how we approach our children. Unfortunately, in western societies we have become too clinical with our children and we have spent a lot of time inval-idating their experiences. As a result, our children learn to dissociate very early in life.

THE CHARACTERISTICS OF DISSOCIATION

If we look to a DSM definition of 'dissociation' it paints a picture of a very unusual and strongly worded definition. In simple terms, dissociation is any of a wide array of experiences from mild detachment from immediate surroundings to more severe detachment from physical and emotional experiences, sense of self, or personal history. The major characteristic of dissociation involves a *detachment* from reality, rather than a *loss* of reality.

It is commonly known that dissociation often occurs in response to trauma, as it provides our system with a protective element that supports us to feel disconnected from traumatic events. In this way it assists us to cope with the reality we are in, especially if that reality is unpleasant. Given everything I have discussed about trauma, you can understand why I say that we all tend to dissociate to some degree – I do it in the gym!

When I'm exercising, my body is often in pain. I just want to disconnect from the reality of my body's experience so I can keep going, because I know that ultimately my body will benefit from the physical exertion, so I want to keep pushing myself. That is dissociation – I am detaching from the reality of what I'm forcing my body to do. If we think over our life experiences, we can recognise that we all tend to dissociate away from discomfort in many and varied situations. It is adaptive and, in many cases, it's a useful tool to support our ability to persevere through discomfort and it supports resilience – but when is it right to teach our children how to do this?

As parents, we begin to teach our infants to dissociate from birth in western cultures. We teach our children to dissociate when we utilise many 'parenting' techniques that have been shown over the past fifty years to effectively elicit from our babies the behaviours that we are expecting from them. It is possible we are actually causing psychological harm in the process.

I discussed controlled crying techniques earlier, this is a favourite of many of the clinics that assist new mothers to learn how to manage their babies' demands. I'm not saying that it isn't effective — it is very effective. However, it is because we 'condition' these children to a particular stimulus/response pairing — we have imposed an external change to nature's normal communication systems. We have taught our children to dissociate.

In many developing nations, where living conditions should result in an inability to thrive, we often see babies who survive horrific conditions due to the fact that their mothers carry them around for the first two years of life. Developmentally, this is an extremely important period for a neonate. The ability to be securely attached to a mother who is available 24/7 to meet their baby's needs, could potentially provide a rationale for their ability to survive in conditions that would otherwise surely result in death. There are obviously many causes of infant mortality, but it makes sense to what we understand about human development to find that a secure attachment would support the developing immune and respiratory systems.

The emotional bond is incredibly powerful, and Pert's research explains a lot of the rationale for why this type of bond would provide the perfect environment for the immune system to become strong.[8] Fogel also provides a rationale for the need for a neonate to be strongly bonded to their primary caregiver, to regulate a range of body systems and support their development.[9] Who knows what would happen to infant mortality rates if western societies provided more support for mothers to keep their babies with them for the majority of their day for the first two years of their life.

There are a range of reasons that the statistics may not be able to definitively support what I am saying here, and the rationale given for what could be seen as a 'causal' link could easily be viewed merely as a 'correlation'. In reality, we can focus on a range of different elements and statistical analyses to argue the pros and cons of my theory, however it is almost impossible to be able to definitively prove this one way or the other. So, all I ask is that we think about it for ourself and make up our own mind about whether or not this seems like it's rational.

The cause of mental health issues

It's important to recognise the issues around attachment, as they are the basis of all of our mental health issues. As I have outlined earlier, the problem with our childhood is there are issues that come up that give rise to significant insecurities about our ability to have our emotional and physical needs met. This is the trouble with trauma. If we don't recognise that this is one of the biggest problems in western societies, and make some active plans to try to change the way we parent, these issues will continue to create more health issues into the future.

We are aware from the ACEs research of the impact of instability and traumatic experiences on the physical body — we are showing the causal link between the psychological and the physiological. The psychological impact begins from the development of the embryo, as our cells respond to their environment. Many of the issues that would lead a child to have traumatic experiences are present around the mother when she is pregnant. They are a product of her socio-economic status and her cultural background and they vary with her level of education. This provides support for a focus on education to afford awareness and clear insight about the linkages between environment and the likely experience of trauma in a child.

It lends itself quite clearly to changes in public policy around a number of issues about supporting families and effective parenting. If we look to our Scandinavian neighbours as good examples of how the focus on the development of families can benefit the whole society, we can see a whole raft of health outcomes that appear to be better than many other western civilisations. They're not perfect, but they are committed to trying to ensure the foundational years for a child are well supported, and this affords the child their best chance at life both physically and emotionally.

If we compare their generalised health data to other countries where children are placed into care from the age of six weeks, we start to see an unwelcome pattern of risk factors for poorer health outcomes. Industrialisation has influenced our effectiveness to raise happy, healthy children. The outcomes of which are starting to become clear.

I can feel the feminists becoming uncomfortable; I really want to make it clear that I am *not* saying women need to be chained to the kitchen and enslaved in domesticity – this isn't the 1950s. However, I think empowered women should be clear that if they choose to have a child, the emphasis being on 'choice', then they probably need to be aware that it is not just an uncomfortable 18 to 24 months of pregnancy and managing the first year.

In reality, a child struggles to cope with big changes in their environment until they are able to more effectively communicate for themselves and start to reason. For these things they usually require language, so they shouldn't have a lot of variety of caregivers until they are about three years old. Even then, they need to experience smaller chunks of alternative care – not being placed in long day care for 10 hours per day from the age of six weeks because mum has to commute an hour each way to an eight-hour work day.

If there is one thing I have learned it is that when we come across information that makes us angry, it has sparked within us a sense of fear or shame. If what I have just outlined above has upset you, I would encourage you to consider why. If you are a parent who had to put your child into long day care and go to work, it may be a sense of shame that you are feeling at my words. Alternatively, you may not have reached this point in your life yet, but recognise that the only way you can afford to have children is by staying at work. I'm really not suggesting that you are doing the wrong thing here. My point is that as a society we need to value motherhood, and western societies do not.

Governments have an important role in putting into place levers that assist us to become the best society we can be, and they have varying policies the world over that are very successful in certain areas. However, I am yet to come across a country that has it *all* sorted. What I am outlining here is merely the recognition that if we truly want to improve the overall health and wellbeing of the human race, we have to be prepared to make hard decisions and educate ourselves to understand how our individual choices impact the collective. We all reside in a community and that community sits within a culture and there are varying levels of government at all levels within the society. We treat mental health as an individual issue, but in reality, our individual health has a direct correlation to our value to the community we reside in.

There are multiple issues that impact us that are external to our nuclear family unit and various societies approach this differently. Rather than trying to determine who is right and who is wrong, what if we could take what appears to be the best of each society and apply it to our situation, if it is possible to do so? After all, the goal here is to create robust communities of healthy individuals who actively connect with family and friends and participate regularly in their community. That should be the goal of every country.

CHAPTER FOUR
RECOVERY

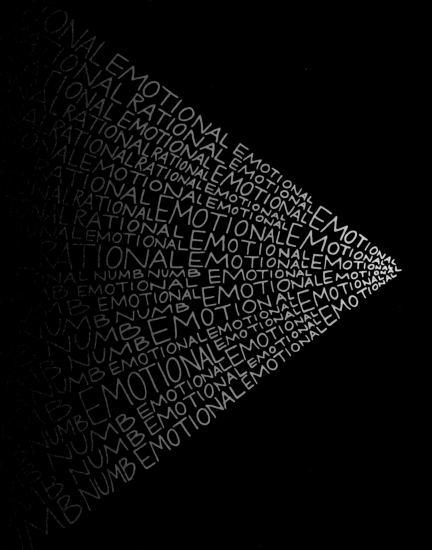

Our Ability To Resolve Our Difficulties
Is Dependent On Our Ability
To Connect With Our Bodies

It's important to recognise that our modern psychological approaches have been built on the back of Descartes's approach to modern medicine; in particular, they have developed mostly in the past 100 years. That's not a whole lot of time in the history of human life. It's important we understand this frame of reference, because there is a tendency among the more intellectual members of the human race to hold the belief that we know all there is to know, which of course, is not possible.

'Nothing in the world is more dangerous than sincere ignorance and conscientious stupidity.'

Martin Luther King Jr

I think this is a particularly important point to clarify, because what I'm about to outline could be perceived as me not supporting the profession to which I belong. Yet, I think this is even more reason to highlight that we do not know everything there is to know about human beings and the essential ingredients to live our best lives. It is a completely individual thing. Yet, we often create a great many rules and draw conclusions that are inflexible, and are unable to open ourselves up to alternative ways of thinking.

MODERN PSYCHOLOGICAL INTERVENTION

It can be really challenging as a psychologist to discuss why I think a lot of modern psychological interventions don't actually help us to resolve these issues. Thankfully, there is also a significant amount of emerging research that supports this perspective.

Most modern psychological techniques teach us to be more self-aware, which is great. In many ways, it helps us to understand how our thinking can affect our feelings and change our behaviours. This level of self-awareness is effective and essential to understanding why we experience difficulties and provides us with strategies to apply different ways of thinking, in the hope we can change how we feel about a variety of situations and how we then behave in response to those triggers.

This is the basic 'triangle' of cognitive behavioural therapy (CBT), and for many people we have greater awareness of the elements at varying points. Some of us are more conscious of our behaviours, and that is the observation point we want to change; others may be aware of their thoughts and want to change those and others want to stop the way they feel. Regardless of where we start, the other two areas closely follow.

The issue with focusing solely on these elements to manage our psychological responses is that it requires 'conscious awareness' of the problem. As such, many people experience years of frustration with certain thoughts, feelings or behaviours, not understanding why they are there, without ever understanding the 'what, why and how' of particular issues.

One of the most commonly used techniques to support psychological intervention is cognitive behavioural therapy. CBT is reported to be one of the most effective psychological treatments, however recent research indicates that the effectiveness of this form of therapy has waned since it was developed 50 years ago.[16] In other research, there is evidence that although CBT is very effective at creating increased self-awareness about the issues that make us feel bad and our ineffective thought patterns, it doesn't appear to afford people the ability to successfully and consistently change their behaviours.[17, 18]

This is often where most psychologists assist people to under-stand the thoughts and feelings that they experience and how they lead to certain behaviours, then provide them the education to bring these things to conscious awareness and strategies to mitigate the impact and/or change the behaviour. This has to be done with 'cognitive awareness' — being aware of our thoughts and how they impact our feelings and result in behavioural change.

There are many benefits to having someone to speak to about the issues that make us feel bad about ourselves. In fact, there is a lot to be said for the benefits of a therapeutic relationship in improving our mood. However, given all of the information I have shared so far, I think it is important to recognise what a lot of psychological treatment supports us to do.

This type of psychological therapy relies on our being able to make the connection to the thought process and actively change it, mostly through diversion techniques or repression. Yes − I am saying that many modern psychological techniques 'teach' people to repress their emotional reactions.

Wait... Doesn't that sound like most modern psychological therapies teach us to dissociate? In my opinion, this is exactly what we learn to do as a result of many of our social interactions, including many therapies.

Let's face it, dissociation is normal − we all do it at certain points in our lives. It's adaptive and can assist us to physically do things in the face of something that would otherwise paralyse us, leading to inaction. I am not saying that it is wrong to assist people to consciously distance themselves from their problems if they are not able to do much to effect change as the problem is outside of their control. However, if we don't recognise the distinction then we will miss the importance of understanding that different types of therapy are effective in resolving different problems.

Most of the focus on therapeutic intervention tends to focus on the 'here and now'. Addressing the issues that are causing us to feel bad about the past and fearful of the future is important, but as we are now aware there are many psychological and physiological reasons for these feelings. The majority of talk therapies are unable to change the behavioural responses that automatically activate in response to triggering of the negative beliefs that develop in response to our early traumatic experiences.

However, there are a number of different therapies that are not focused on our ability to be cognitively aware of what the issue is and consciously make adjustments to our thoughts. There are therapies that allow us to make adjustments at the subconscious level, but this is the 'great unknown' in terms of how we control our perspectives. As a result, the subconscious frightens many of us, including many psychological therapists.

It is human nature to want to be in control of our situation and not be taken outside of our comfort zone. Psychologists, as a profession, are no different. Although, usually people who are drawn into the profession are there because they genuinely seek to help people and they don't like to see people in emotional pain. As a result, some of the therapeutic processes that address things that are stored in our unconscious mind are perceived to be less predictable and this creates uncertainty. For many therapists, it's this uncertainty that makes them feel uncomfortable and so they will often stick to therapeutic processes that are more 'conscious', even if those processes do not appear to be as effective or efficient.

I highlight this because it is important to recognise that psychologists are ultimately people too — they have flaws just like any other human being. If they have studied human nature, it just means that they are humans with (hopefully) a better understanding of human behaviour and enhanced communication skills. However, they are not magical or mystical and they can't possibly all be 'all' things to 'all' people. Sometimes they get it wrong.

I liken the majority of contemporary therapy to psychoeducation and awareness raising, coupled with learned strategies to combat the feelings and behaviours in a controlled and conscious way. It can be effective, but it's also hard work. I often have clients who come to me in frustration that they understand what's going on and why they 'react' to certain triggers, but they're tired of feeling like they are constantly having to consciously fight with themselves.

So how do we do it better?

'The only thing more dangerous than ignorance is arrogance.'

Albert Einstein

Resolving trauma

I often describe the way trauma impacts our system as similar to an old party treat called a 'frog in the pond'. In essence, it is a dessert made with green jelly, and each small bowl has a chocolate frog set in the jelly.

I say that when a traumatic event occurs, we make jelly. We pour the jelly crystals and the hot water into a glass bowl, but we need to allow the jelly time to cool down before we can position the chocolate frog in place. Too early and it will melt; too long and the jelly will crack; but once it is correctly in place we can't get it out without breaking everything. It's jelly in a glass bowl – so it's transparent.

The chocolate frog is representative of the traumatic event. We can take that bowl of jelly to every therapist in town, we understand what the chocolate frog is about and how it got there. We can turn that bowl upside down, but still it won't budge. We can talk about the problem with many people and we can understand how it got stuck, but talk therapies don't allow us to change the way it makes us feel.

Gaining clarity

So, how do they help us to resolve it? Primarily, they assist us to gain clarity about what the chocolate frog represents for us, and can help us see that we have a lot of other things to focus on rather than this frog. However, if we really want to just have the frog gone from our life because we feel like we've grown up and now prefer pavlova, it's not an effective solution.

In many ways, modern therapy teaches us to try to tolerate the impact of our emotional experiences. It's not been an unreasonable approach to take, given that we didn't have any other way to manage except to try to learn to 'cope' with the feelings. However, our understanding of many things in science has come a very long way, and I don't think modern medicine or therapy approaches have moved as quickly.

There are many and varied reasons for this – arguably, psychological ones! However, what we often find is that it is the tendency to be firm in our 'beliefs' that actually creates bigger problems. In essence, as human beings we tend to hold tight to a particular way of looking at the world if we have had experiences that confirm a particular approach seems effective.

To try to help us understand what I'm getting at, let's look at the life of Charles Darwin. He proposed a theory about human evolution that he adamantly defended until his much later life, when he said that maybe he hadn't actually taken *all* the evidence into account.

This is representative of a common psychological phenomenon known as 'confirmation bias', and it's based on the fact that when we have to strongly defend a position we have taken, we often fight harder for that position, and hold much tighter to it, than if we had been more open to the perspective that other people are able to form a different opinion.

There are many reasons we form cognitive biases; they do actually assist our system to make rational and effective decisions and there are *a lot* of them. Think of them like little 'short cuts' that our brain has set up in a complex system that allows us to quickly categorise our experiences — but sometimes we get it wrong.

What is also interesting is that if we realise we 'got it wrong' to begin with, we create a situation of cognitive dissonance, a psychological phenomenon in which we hold two or more opposing beliefs, values or ideas about something. Our brain doesn't like it, and it causes us quite a lot of psychological discomfort. In order to resolve the discomfort, we almost 'oversubscribe' to the new way of thinking. It's like in order to change our first opinion, we have to become a 'champion' of the new cause.

As a result, we will find that when we have developed strong beliefs about a particular issue, we will hold tighter to those beliefs if they are ever challenged. If we have felt the need to defend those beliefs at any point, our commitment to them becomes stronger. This is the basis for all of the extremism in the world, and it manifests in many areas of our society, between cultures, and particularly strongly in mainstream religions.

This is why I wrote my first book *Define Your Inner Diva* as I was trying to help people to understand that the reason we can't live the happy life we really want has its basis in how we feel about ourselves. We think that we're unhappy because of our relationships, our dissatisfaction with our work or with our approach to our health. However, in that book I highlight why all of these elements actually have their basis in our inability to accept ourselves and what people need to do to understand and resolve those issues.

In this book I have taken you into more detail about 'why' trauma has such a big impact on our physiological bodies. In essence, we need to resolve the underlying negative belief system that we have formed as a result of our traumatic experiences, in order to be able to have the best chance of being able to live our best life, feeling satisfied and being healthy. I wanted to expand on what I had written in my first book to broaden out the implications of why we need to recognise the impact of trauma on our physical bodies, not just in our psychological thinking.

Rather than reiterating here about the strategies that you can undertake to resolve your underlying negative beliefs; I would encourage you to refer back to my first book as a 'workbook' to assist you to resolve the issues. I'm even going to give you a special discount to enable you to grab an ebook copy for only $2.99. If you head over to Amazon.com and search for 'Define Your Inner Diva' you will see that the Kindle version is already discounted for you.

Suffice to say that there are several types of therapies that address the subconscious and provide ways to treat those automated patterns of thoughts, feelings and behaviour in ways that are not just 'band-aids', but truly resolve the issues fully.

I suggest you try an EMDR Therapist or a Resource State Therapist – there is a link to the various international organisations on my website (kerryannhoward.com) or you can ask Google. The great thing about these types of therapies is that they are effective and efficient forms that actually change the underlying beliefs you hold about yourself, and in this way, we are most likely to be able resolve long-standing beliefs. We want to engage in a therapeutic process that will allow us to 'heal' the negative belief system, not just use a band-aid solution.

A substantial body of research shows that adverse life experiences contribute to both psychological and biomedical pathology. EMDR Therapy is an empirically validated treatment for trauma, and other mental health issues. Twenty-four randomised controlled trials support the positive effects of EMDR Therapy in the treatment of emotional trauma and other adverse life experiences. Numerous other evaluations document that EMDR therapy provides relief from a variety of somatic complaints.[19] There is significant research that demonstrates the physiological benefits of bilateral stimulation that EMDR Therapy utilises.

During an EMDR Therapy session, you recall traumatic or triggering experiences in brief doses while the therapist directs your eye movements or provides some other form of bilateral stimulation – such as auditory or tactile stimulation (BLS). The research provides evidence that supports the preference of eye movement over other types of input as it appears to be the most consistent in providing effective long-term outcomes.

There are a variety of theoretical underpinnings to why EMDR Therapy works, and if you are interested you can find significant amounts of information about it – but the main thing to note is that it works and it has had a lot of research that provides evidence of its effectiveness.

Alan Fogel reviews EMDR Therapy in his book *Body Sense* and identifies that it heightens embodied self-awareness, allowing a person to be present with current emotional states while recalling previously suppressed emotions and feelings.[9]

Fogel's book is focused on the importance of connecting to the self through our bodies:

Embodied self-awareness is as fundamental to health and survival as breathing and eating... The loss of embodied self-

awareness at any time in life is debilitating... Embodied self-awareness is easily lost whilst growing up in technological societies, by cumulative deprivation, or by sudden traumas... Embodied self-awareness must be actively maintained, cultivated, taught and renewed to sustain well-being.[*]

Fogel not only reviews EMDR Therapy but provides an understanding for why the eyes are significant in processing experiences. He refers to the involvement of extraocular muscles behind our eyes in the face of a threat — they tense in a way that restricts the gaze and consequently leads to facial muscle tension and eye strain. When we are faced with a threat our gaze usually becomes fixed and darting, vigilant in trying to assess our options — fight, flight or freeze.

Eye movement in EMDR Therapy is similar to the flexible patterns of eye movement that we observe with REM sleep or other situations in which we feel safe and relaxed. Fogel goes on to highlight that the extraocular muscles are linked to patterns of muscle tension in the face, head, tongue, neck, chest, abdomen and pelvis. In fact, they are a primary activator for our neuromuscular system. Eye movement can evoke referred pain and tension but also relaxation in muscles throughout the body.[9] In this way, EMDR Therapy allows our emotional processing to occur while our body is experiencing an action that is linked to being calm and safe and the arousal in the face of activation becomes extinguished.

I didn't understand all of these physiological linkages when I first engaged in EMDR Therapy — long story short, I had an accident. When I was 28, I was hit by a bus as a pedestrian and lived to tell the tale. Surprisingly, I only suffered minor injuries but the trauma took its toll on my mental health. I suffered Post Traumatic Stress Disorder (PTSD) and secondary Depression. I tried to resolve things myself; I had always been a pretty strong and independent person — but I couldn't fix this.

---

[*]   *Body Sense,* page 15.

I saw a psychologist, and thankfully she had trained in EMDR Therapy. This is a big part of the reason why I later became an EMDR therapist, because I knew from personal experience that it really works! In my experience, EMDR Therapy isn't just a band-aid solution, helping to repress things again — it really heals.

I have worked with clients using EMDR Therapy for over a decade and I am constantly amazed by the effectiveness of the therapy. There are very strong links between our physical bodies and the processing of our traumatic experiences — when we are working with EMDR Therapy we are always linking the traumatic experience to where it is felt in the body — which is why it helps to increased embodied self-awareness.

When we consider the opportunities to resolve our physiological and psychological challenges, there is no doubt that our ability to do this is dependent on our ability to connect with our bodies and allow ourselves to express our emotions and experiences.

JUDGEMENT

I once wrote a chapter for a book called *Better Business, Better Life, Better World*. Along with many of my fellow members of B1G1 — Business For Good, I was asked if I could outline what I wanted my grandchildren to know about life, business and the world. I have provided my contribution in the appendix.

What's interesting is I wrote that nearly four years ago, and my perspective hasn't changed. In fact, it grows stronger every day that I see more unrest in the world. I've stopped watching the news because I hear enough 'bad news' from my clients about the atrocities of modern humanity; I don't need to have that reinforced in front of my eyes every night! I'm really no worse off for it.

I used to say I wanted to eliminate 'judgement' from the world. However, I came to realise that judgement is essential to our ability to grow as human beings, and we use it to assess our situation every day, in many and varied ways. It's actually what helps to keep us safe — it's the part of our brain that tells our amygdala to calm down when we jump at a stick because we thought it was a snake. We need to utilise judgement to manage ourselves and those we are responsible for. What we don't need judgement for is to unnecessarily assess the actions of our fellow humans.

It's not very clear exactly 'when' we started judging others — but it has to have been thousands and thousands of years ago, because our ancient history tells us about all of the varying 'conquerors' in the world. Dictators and rulers who decided they wanted what someone else had, and they were going to make sure they obtained it — no matter the cost.

This approach actually predates modern religions, so the fact that most of the religious writings in the world talk about 'do not covet thy brother's wife' also implies that we should not seek to take something someone else has. In fact, going right back to the 'Garden of Eden' or whatever other creation story we may subscribe to (or not), there is a sense of doing what is 'right', and the fact that we might desire something which doesn't belong to us was morally understood to be wrong. This has been the basis of modern religious teachings for centuries, as has the notion of not 'judging' others. Yet somewhere along the line, these basic moral codes have been lost.

I go back to the point that dictatorships and conquering other nations has happened since the evolution of humans, but I believe that over time it has changed from being based in the belief we need to retain that which belongs to us. At some point, desire overcame some natural born leaders and they instigated actions that led to a continuous and unrelenting pursuit for retribution. As a result, we now regularly see world leaders vying for their position at the top of the chain of command — dictators in chief who demonstrate ever escalating narcissistic behaviours and manipulate the masses into believing they're 'justified' in their acts of retribution. Yet most of these world leaders espouse a belief in religion that is grounded in showing mercy, love and acceptance.

Perhaps I am being too hopeful that as we are able to educate more and more humans, this improved awareness will result in an acceptance that people are able to make their own judgements about what is right for their own lives, and as long as it doesn't impact on my life and I don't impact on yours, we can live quite harmoniously together. If we stopped trying to vie for 'top dog', we might be able to find harmony in the pack – natural leadership because a person has lived a life in open-minded acceptance of the right of the individual to choose their own path.

When I think of the world's leading influencers who have demonstrated these types of behaviours, I think of people like the Dalai Lama, Gandi, Mother Teresa, and for different reasons, Nostradamus. I'm not saying these people are perfect humans completely without judgement, but they are selfless human beings who have lived their life with a purpose – to improve humanity for all of us. The truly selfless do not operate from a place of ego, they just share their insights and experiences, and hope to learn from others and allow others to learn from them. This is truly the 'universe' at its energetic best – shining light to humanity that there is a different way to do things.

It is not surprising that my perspective on life is influenced by my recognition that we are human beings who are made up of energy. A conglomeration of cells, brought together for the benefit of each of those cells, due to the fact that our cells have learned they can achieve more if they stick together. Through connection, our cells are able to achieve more. Which is why, ultimately, when we break it down – a single cell is the primary basis on which human life is able to be built.

I am not a biologist. I would encourage you to read the books of those who are – such as *The Biology of Belief* by Dr Bruce Lipton[20] and *Molecules of Emotion* by Dr Candace Pert.[8] I found in their research much of the validation for the perspective I am sharing with you here about the mind and body connection and why we need to open our minds to the fact that we still have so much to learn about ourselves.

How our bodies adapt

In particular, Dr Bruce Lipton provides a very clear explanation of the fact that, as human beings, we are 'energy' beings, but we treat ourselves as if we are 'chemical' beings. His perspective on cells and how they communicate really helped me to understand how changes in our cellular functioning are strongly tied to our emotions, and how these can be altered by our beliefs. His research also explains how we inherit biological information through our DNA, but that it is not as 'fixed' as some people believe.

The way I describe our biological inheritance is it's like we are given a blueprint of the outline for a house in our DNA, so we are given the structure of it — it could be a six-room house. However, our environment can adjust how that house looks, and over time we can adjust our DNA strands based on our experiences. This is also reflected in the process of neuroplasticity.

Dr Lipton talks about cells and how, at the most basic level, they are like mini-humans, single-celled organisms that formed relationships with other 'like' cells for the benefit of all cells. In this way, our most basic biological element performs much like we do, as an organism made up of billions of cells who collaborate with other organisms for the benefit of all those 'like' organisms.

Interestingly, he also breaks down the elements of a cell and aligns the varying parts to their counterparts in the human organism. He describes how the cell nucleus was often thought to represent the cell's brain. However, through research they have shown that the nucleus actually appears to be the reproductive centre of the cell. If we remove the cell nucleus, the cell will take approximately two months to die. Without reproductive capability, the cell eventually dies, but the effect is not immediate.

Through his research, Dr Lipton was able to demonstrate it is actually the cell membrane that is the real 'brain' of the cell, and he tried (unsuccessfully) to get biologists to rename it the 'membrain'. Interestingly, I take this notion one step further, and I think we can refer to it as the 'memory-brain', as this is how information from our ancestors is passed on, through the cellular imprint. This includes the imprinting of their traumatic experiences on our membrains.

Nature versus nurture

This concept is an incredibly important one to understand, because in trauma therapy we are very clear about understanding that we can experience 'intergenerational trauma'. However, many psychologists have considered it a phenomenon that was related to the 'nurture' component of our psychological makeup. In essence, this implies our parents conditioned us to respond in a specific way to a stimulus based on their own experience – their fears and shame. However, I believe Dr Lipton's approach about the cell membrane being the 'membrain' is the key to this mystery, and shows there is a 'memory-brain' component to the membrane. The genetic encoding of trauma is also part of our blueprint.

There are various areas of emerging neuroscientific research about why this is a more likely explanation for intergenerational trauma, however I am not ignoring the fact that there are some who would prefer to think of it as a 'nurture' rather than a 'nature' explanation, but I believe both elements are at play.

I recall a story of a friend who noted an unusual phenomenon about how he slept. He used to roll his head from side to side in his sleep, and he thought it was a bit odd. He was aware he had done this all his life, and didn't know why, but he almost rocked his head in his sleep.

He happened to be speaking to his mother about this curiosity when he was in his mid-30s, and his mother reported that she knew exactly what he was talking about as his father also did the same thing in his sleep. Intrigued by this, he approached his father and explained how he rocked his head in his sleep, and his mother had said his father also did this, and he wondered if his father had any insight into why.

Interestingly, this man's father had been a baby when he was put in a POW camp in Germany during the Second World War. He had lived there from the age of one to four years. His father looked at him and said: 'Yes... I do that. When I was in the POW camp, I had to rock my head at night to stop the rats chewing at my ears. I just never really stopped the habit.' My friend was amazed that he had inherited this behaviour in the absence of any direct threat to his own ears. Perhaps unsurprisingly, his niece also rocks her head in her sleep, in the absence of any ongoing active threat.

However, with what we understand about how our cells respond to their environment, we can approach this with an entirely different perspective. This man's father had developed a process for avoiding a negative impact, and he had performed it effectively for so long that it impacted his 'normal' processes – it became his new 'norm'.

As such, it became 'set' in his brain as an effective avoidance strategy. So much so that even long after the 'threat' was no longer present, his physical response was still active. The strategy became the new 'set point' for his brain about how to avoid the threat of rats harming his ears, even without the presence of the 'actual' threat. This had then encoded itself on his DNA, and was passed through to his son and his granddaughter, who then performed the same behaviour without any conscious decision, source or rationale.

In a psychological sense, we are aware that what this man developed in his childhood was 'operant conditioning'. You may be aware of the Pavlov's Dog experiments that prove how we can create an automated response as a reaction to a specific trigger. What many psychologists are unaware of is that due to the environmental response of our cellular functioning, if the conditioning isn't extinguished, it would leave a permanent imprint on the DNA of an individual.

In terms of intergenerational trauma, this helps us to understand how the 'nature' element of the traumatic imprint is passed on. It makes perfect sense when we consider as humans have evolved, each generation stores the new biological information that is applicable to the environment we have adapted to, and brings with it changes that support our adaption into the future.

It also helps us to understand how it is that we are able to inherit a range of psychological issues. Anyone who has been diagnosed with a mental health condition at any point in their life will know that the GP will ask about any family history of mental health issues. This is because the medical fraternity are aware of the genetic predisposition we have based on the experiences of our parents, however they seem to believe that this is a 'set' blueprint — they are not yet aware that the biological response is highly susceptible to change based on our environment. This is the concept of neuroplasticity. Many in the medical profession still hold on to the notion that genetic inheritance is fixed — we just need to learn how to cope with it. However, what emerging research implies is that *nothing* is fixed — we can change *everything* about how we respond to stimulus — both physical and psychological.

This has been a ground-breaking concept for me in my development as a professional over many years, but it also made so much sense that I just can't put people into a definitive 'box' anymore. I can assist people to understand how their life experiences have come to be, and this may be in part due to some level of genetic inheritance, but I no longer believe the issues we think are 'biological' — the implication being that this means they can't be changed — are absolutely correct. I believe we could even change really 'complex' mental health conditions like bipolar or schizophrenia, and I believe our current environment is responsible for the rise of conditions like ADHD — which has a highly genetic predisposition but is exacerbated by our modern living conditions and the pace at which we live our lives, including the availability of technology. Let's be real — we no longer have to retain information; we have technology at

our fingertips, and Google tells us anything it wants us to know...
And therein lies the danger.

I find it fascinating that this is so challenging for people to accept,
yet we are aware of many other physiological processes that adapt
in response to changes in conditions. Think of what happens when
we 'diet' — we all know eventually our metabolism adjusts to the
change in conditions and our weight loss will slow down. So, in
response to this, many people have turned to intermittent fasting,
with amazing success. This is due to the fact that our physical body
is unable to achieve homeostasis, because as soon as it seems to adjust
to the new regime, we change it and starve it, so it can't get settled
on the expectation of a specific caloric intake.

We know our bodies do this in response to other extreme
intermittent activities, like exercise or temperature. We know high
intensity interval training (HIIT) can provide some fast and unexpected benefits in terms of muscle gain and mitochondria release,
which is good for our brains. Also, we know moving from hot
environments to cold environments can provide the body with a
variety of benefits. I discuss these approaches in more detail later,
but suffice to say that our bodies do respond to unexpected experiences as they get 'used' to new things fairly quickly.

In addition to the changes we see from changing what impacts
our bodies, we can also observe changes in our physiological
response when we start feeding our bodies with things that it
doesn't normally get — like long-term medications.

Most people will have had an experience, or know someone who
has had the experience, of starting on a longer term medication and
needing to make adjustments for this over time, as the body adapts to
the new chemical being regularly fed into it. The medical profession
understands this is 'normal', and they will work with their patients
to review medication and make adjustments until the patient appears
to be receiving the intended benefit. In the same way, they will
advise slowly easing off a long-term medication so as to allow the
body time to adjust. Our body adjusts to the new 'set point' as we are

biologically programmed to try to maintain homeostasis – which is the tendency towards a relatively stable equilibrium between interdependent elements, especially those maintained physiologically.

It should come as no surprise then that we are able to make physiological and psychological adjustments over time. Certain therapies facilitate these adjustments more effectively than others, however you should consult your doctor before commencing any program.

JUDGEMENTAL? OR MISGUIDED LOYALTY?

I think it's an important segue at this point to tell you that I myself have spent many years holding fast to strong beliefs and opinions. Many people think that because of the way I speak about things with conviction, I'm tied to a particular belief system. However, the experiences of my life do not support this perspective.

Interestingly, culturally I have a lot of Scottish and Irish DNA. In fact, my mother is a Macleod and the family motto is 'Hold Fast' – so I will lay the blame on my genetic imprint for this part of the perspective that people have of me! Thankfully, I think I have enough DNA from the Druids to be able to trust in myself and my own intuition, so much so that I don't need to apologise for the portrayal of my insight and wisdom.

However, I haven't always been so open to different ways of thinking. I was born into a Catholic household and educated in a Catholic school for many of my influential early childhood years. Then my mother became a 'born again' Christian when I was in early high school, and she managed to lure me into the Church by engaging my natural, and insatiable, curious nature. In many ways, my teen years were strongly influenced by that Christian judgement, but I never felt accepted by anyone. I have always felt 'different' to my peers. I believe those years of attempted indoctrination by the dogma of religious extremism ultimately did me a favour; it made me more aware of the varied moral values of society and very clear about the hypocritical actions of human beings — those who profess certain beliefs, but their behaviour belies those beliefs.

I actually committed time at the tender age of 18 to become a modern-day 'missionary' — but in truth, I think I was just fascinated by the idea of world travel! I was never very good at 'witnessing' — the act of door knocking and bothering people in their own homes to try to influence them to come around to a different way of thinking.

I still remember that when I had to 'report' about my activities in the conversion of the world, one heart at a time, I couldn't be honest about the fact that I really just didn't hold enough conviction to be any good at door knocking. In fact, what usually happened is I would knock on a few doors on day one in an area, and I would make a new friend. Then I would spend every day 'witnessing' to my new friend over coffee. We called this 'lifestyle evangelism', but really, I was just making connections.

I like to think that those 'friends' would still recall my visits with a smile on their face. The larrikin 'Aussie girl' who showed up on their doorstep and was happy to talk about life's challenges over a cuppa. My real love was for helping people, by accepting them for who they were, not by trying to change them to some notion of who I conceived they should be.

My commitment to this religious organisation was, not surprisingly, cut short. You see, my body knew things that my mind was not able to fathom at this point. The organisation I was volunteering for provided my board and lodgings, in return for the work I did to support their missionary acts. However, I had very little control over my circumstances in that place. As things became more uncomfortable for me and I felt more and more control slipping through my fingers, my body started to respond to the things my mind wasn't rationalising. Not surprisingly, I became quite ill.

This is a good example of what we call in psychological circles 'somatic symptoms'. The problem is many people believe 'somatic' means 'fake' — somehow deliberately created from the subconscious recesses of our mind to appear as physical, but it's just 'all in our head!' These days, I understand this extremely well and there is nothing manufactured about it.

I developed stomach ulcers — I was 19 years old! I was drinking Gaviscon three times a day and really struggling with my stomach. Over several months, these issues became more and more problematic, and ultimately the stress impact was so severe that I needed to find a way to return home — only seven months into my two-year commitment to this organisation.

So, if it wasn't just in my head, what was actually happening?

Somatic symptoms

Many of you will be aware that we will experience issues in our gut when our fears are raised. It's actually neurological when confronted with a threat; our amygdala sends the message to our gut that we need to 'fight or flee', and depending on which we need to do, our body will usually bind itself together or evacuate the system. There is good reason we colloquially use the term 'I s*%t myself!' in response to fear — although maybe that's just Australians. Our body will take control of our gut, in order to ensure we can take the appropriate action to save ourselves.

Interestingly, our intestines and our brain actually develop from the same part of the neural tube when we are only an embryo. The intestine even looks like our brain! There are many of the same cells in our gut as there are in our brain; in fact, we now know that most of the serotonin we produce (the neurotransmitter that is predominantly believed to control our feelings of happiness) is produced in our gut — not our brain!

There is more and more science emerging every day about the impact of gut health on our experiences of depression and anxiety. When we think about it a bit more laterally, it makes perfect sense that the cellular functioning of the gut has a significant influence on our brains. Antidepressants are swallowed as a pill that is absorbed into our gut, and they impact how our brain feels. Hello!? Are we really so naive as to think it is somehow a one-way system? Impenetrable from one side, but completely open on the other? Many pharmaceutical companies would have us believe this because it keeps their profits up and their shareholders happy.

In any case, my stomach was responding to the constant feelings of being different and not belonging, and the lack of acceptance from the women I was forced to share a home with, and I was powerless to do anything about it. I coped for the first few months because I had an 'escape' − I was the only one authorised by the organisation to drive the car that was afforded to our household, so I could get away any time I wanted to.

After a few months though, my fellow household members were making plans to also gain authority to drive the car, and my escape route started to come under threat. So, of course, my physical symptoms got worse and worse the more that my opportunity for freedom came under threat. Fight or flight! I wasn't able to fight; the organisation had rules and obligations and I had willingly signed up to those. So I found a little way to escape, and that allowed me to obtain some balance in my life as I was able to regularly connect with a group of people who found my 'difference' refreshing and interesting − they made me feel valued for the first time in my life.

It comes as no surprise that as my freedom started to look like it was going to be taken away from me, my stomach started to do its own little revolt. My gut was responding to the fact I felt trapped and I couldn't fight; I was losing my opportunity to escape when I wanted to, and if I became fenced in and froze, the next biologically rational point in the face of the threat was death.

Now, rationally, had I been a little older and wiser, I may have been able to find an alternative solution to this problem. However, I had been raised by a very strong, independent single mother, and I had learned from a very young age that I had to rely on myself to get out of situations. I tried to look at a number of options, but they would only let me 'out' if I was returning home after my two-year commitment had been fulfilled. Even with my ever-looming health issues, they would only offer to relocate me to another country in support of the organisation.

To my mind, which was focused on fleeing, the idea of being in a different country, away from the only social supports I had ever known that I felt accepted me and therefore provided me with a vital connection that sustained life as I knew it, was completely off the table! Imagine being in a foreign country with these already difficult health problems and then having to learn a new language and potentially finding myself on the 'outer' again. I couldn't take that risk. I was like a deer in the headlights — assessing *every* pathway out. However, I was trapped — my visa was linked to the organisation, and I was not able to work elsewhere to earn the money I needed to support myself there, or to earn the money for a return ticket home.

Guardian angels

In the end, the universe provided me with a couple of guardian angels. One from within my new social group, my 'family' of choice, and the other was the woman within the organisation who had filled the role of my 'mother figure' while I was there. Between them, they paid for my plane fare home. Andy and Carole — two people I will never forget for their kindness and generosity. I hope the universe rewarded them for their 'pay it forward' act of kindness, for I was never able to actually repay them. By the time I was in a position to do so, I was unable to locate either of them.

When I returned home, my Mum had decided to move back to the city of our birth — Melbourne. Here my health issues managed to settle down again, and I found myself still drawn to the Church, trying to find myself a group to connect with that would make me feel accepted.

Again, I struggled to fit in. I will never forget the point I decided organised religion was not really for me. I was 19 years old. I had been attending the same Church for about nine months, and I had the opportunity to make my Debut. Debutante Balls were not common, but were still a bit of a social tradition which seemed like fun to my curious mind. There had been a wild moment in my seventeenth year in which I had thought I would marry (I blame the Church!) – but the notion of being twirled around a dance floor in a pretty white dress was super appealing to me. So, I decided I would do it.

Interestingly, it was this decision that would give rise to my clarity about the judgement of others and when it was displaced. You see, to be presented at the debutante ball I had to find someone to partner me and we had to attend dance lessons for about eight weeks. This was a major event held at the Melbourne Town Hall – I do have a habit of deciding if I'm going to do something, I like to do a good job of it!

My partner for this event was one of the young men from our youth group, a guy called Derek who was just a friend. Our decision to do the Debutante Ball had nothing to do with our commitment to the Church, nor did it impact our faith in any way... It just meant that instead of attending Church twice on Sunday, we were only attending the evening service for the period we were practising for the ball. But for some reason, senior members of the Church leadership didn't see it this way. My mother was spoken to, and I was 'counselled' for my lack of commitment to the Church and my responsibility for leading my friend Derek astray!

Now, if there is one thing, I know about myself, it's that I have no tolerance for injustice, and this was unjust. There was no validity to their opinion about my choice to take part in a community activity. Their assessment of my motives and my influence over Derek was completely irrational and not based in any element of truth. Instead, they were imposing a biased perspective, passing judgement, and demanding I submit to the authority of the Church leadership and stop what I was doing and repent for the damage I was causing Derek.

It was a blatant attempt at disempowering me as a woman and labelling me with the responsibility for leading a poor young man astray with my feminine wiles... It was one of the most disgusting displays of chauvinistic oppression I have seen in my life. And I was not going to stand for it!

I told them what I thought of their misplaced judgements, and walked out of that Church, not to set foot inside one again for about 10 years.

Extreme empowerment creates disconnection

This did a couple of things to me — I felt empowered that I had stood up for myself, but at the same time I found myself alone, without connection and again in a place where I felt rejected. I struggled for quite a while after that. Around this time my Mum had been offered a job in a regional town and she moved away, and I ended up moving into a flat by myself — more disconnection.

Not surprisingly, my mood deteriorated significantly. I reached out to try to form connections in other areas, through colleagues and social interests, but I really struggled. This was also a period where I looked to fill the void with a boyfriend, but due to how I was feeling about myself, I was only attracting people who were not treating me well. What I didn't understand about myself then, was that it made sense I wasn't able to find a good intimate relationship. You see, I didn't like me very much, so how could I draw someone to me who cared for me if I didn't feel deserving of the connection? It was a very difficult time...

I became quite ill in this period. I managed to pick up what they called the 'Bali Flu' — it was a terrible flu that kept me bedridden for about five days and added to my feelings of loneliness and isolation.

I reached a point during this period — after feeling rejected by yet another young man — that I was so low I had decided there was no point in living. I was distraught, and decided I was just going to take my own life. I still remember driving my car along the freeway thinking about how I could have a crash that was sure to kill me, but no matter which way I looked at it I couldn't see a way to do it that would be sure to do the job, especially without putting anybody else at risk. So, I decided I needed another way.

I thought about some other options, and rested on an overdose as being most likely to give me what I felt I so strongly wanted but not likely to cause any major issues if it failed (such a girly way to think about it!). However, when I returned to my little flat the only medication I had was the contraceptive pill and Panadol! Neither of these was going to do the job... I broke at that point — crying and berating myself for the fact that I couldn't even kill myself properly! I found myself in a heap in the bath, unable to move or do much except cry.

I now understand this was my child part — at this point I had moved from the protector who was trying to take the ultimate decision to protect my system by ending the pain in the only way I knew how — to the child who just felt unwanted, unloved and alone.

My cat jumped onto the end of the bath and sat looking at me in my crying foetal position in the water, and he was miaowing at me in a way that said, 'What are you doing?' Of course, the child in me responded to the love of my cat — it wasn't much, but it was something. It was enough connection to make me feel someone cared about whether I lived or died... And in that moment, it was enough to bring me to a place where I could get out of the bath and go to bed, where I snuggled with my cat and cried myself to sleep.

Things looked different the next morning. I had turned a corner in some ways because I had decided that if I couldn't kill myself, I had to find a better way to live. I made some big decisions then; I got a second job to fill in my time, and I did a course that would help me become more empowered.

I took back control of my life.

I empowered myself through education, and I facilitated new connections in my life. I spent a lot of time reflecting on something I used to say to my Mum about finding a new relationship in her life: 'Mum, he's not going to come and knock on the door like a present tied up in a bow saying "here I am" — you have to put yourself out there so you can find each other!'

So, I took a piece of my own advice and I got busy. Soon after that, I met my future husband and life took yet another turn.

I learned through this difficult period that life was going to throw challenges my way, whether I liked it or not. I needed to try to educate myself to handle those challenges as best I could. If I wanted my life to be different, I was the only one who could make it so.

God helps those who help themselves!

This has been a motto I have held with me since my late teens, and it has served me well.

RESILIENCE OR REPRESSION?

Most psychologists would see what I did at this point in my life as a good demonstration of my resilience – my ability to pick myself up by the bootstraps, dust myself off and move forward. I showed strength and this is something that our western society values. In reality, I just managed to repress my feelings of worthlessness behind my ability to keep busy. I also used my focus on continuous improvement to make me feel that I was able to have some control over my outcomes and I set about trying to 'prove myself' to the world. As it turned out, this wasn't necessarily all negative, but it really didn't do anything to resolve the underlying feelings of not being good enough that had plagued me over my life. It just gave me a way to push it onto the back-burner for a while.

You see, I still hadn't been able to address the needs of the little girl inside of me who was looking for unconditional love... And it would be many years before I would be able to truly help her.

I spent the next 21 years still trying to prove myself and fill the void of my own lack of self-acceptance or feeling loveable. I had major milestones at the seven-year cycle points in my life – I remember the first time I was able to look back over my life and see those points – like beacons flashing in the dark, clear markers of major life change points. They were all there:

- **7:** when I first felt the full burden of responsibility for my parents' marriage breakdown

- **14:** when I was ultimately rejected by my father — definitively

- **21:** when I married for the first time — I thought I had found love and acceptance

- **28:** when I was hit by a bus as a pedestrian and really started to understand who I was as a human being and develop some self-awareness and self-acceptance

- **35:** when I married for the second time — I thought I had found protection and support for growth (mid-life renewal and rebirth — we know we haven't got the life we want and we want a 'do over' so we refocus and begin again)

- **42:** when I finally became a fully qualified psychologist

- **49:** when I put all the pieces of the puzzle together and was able to share this with you in this book.

At varying points over my life I have experienced abandonment and rejection, but I have equally experienced love, joy, peace and connection. The good and the bad. And as I have aged, I have continued to experience a greater level of insight and self-acceptance. Not because my life got easier, but because I have always practised what I preach, and I've done a lot of therapy work over the last 21 years! Therapy that worked.

I'm not saying I'm perfect — far from it. But I have a level of self-acceptance and love for who I am as a person so that I'm not easily swayed by the opinions of those around me. I actually really like who I am as a person and I am accepting that not everyone is going to like me, and that's honestly okay. I can sometimes have self-doubt, although it is much rarer now. The only place it tends to still strongly influence me is with my family or my partner. However, I have a much more self-aware and more manageable way of handling any negative feelings that might pop up on occasion with those closest to me, but it really is miniscule in comparison to the inadequacies I used to feel about myself.

As a result of this new found 'self-acceptance', my interpersonal connections have grown. My willingness to be open and honest about who I am as a human being has significantly expanded my social connections. I have a much wider group of friends now than I have ever had at any point before in my life. The consistent feedback I get from those people is they are drawn to my openness and genuine acceptance of others, without judgement.

It's interesting because I never seek that from people. It's quite strange; many people will look at me, and because of the way I present myself they can make judgements about my own ego or self-importance (I have bright pink hair). However, anyone who moves past that initial perspective with an open mind will often report they don't actually get that feeling from me at all.

Don't get me wrong: when I was young I held strong opinions and would engage people about them. However, I quickly learned I wasn't interested in trying to persuade others, but I was rigid in not allowing them to persuade me! Almost dogmatic, but in a passive-aggressive way. As I have aged, I am more open to sharing my perspectives and hearing the views of others, in mutual respect for their perspective.

CURIOUS QUESTIONING

That's why I often talk about exploring concepts with 'curious questioning'. When I am engaged in an intellectual conversation about concepts or perspectives on life, I see it as holding a space between myself and the others involved, into which we can place our perspective for the observation of others. I liken it to playing open-handed poker — laying our cards on the table because we're happy with our hand, rather than observing and manipulating to take from others what we want. In this way, we are all holding a space in mutual respect for those we are connecting with.

You can imagine when we do this the energy around that connection is much more positive and engaging than if everyone at the table was trying to dominate or usurp the others involved. This is why when we eliminate the judgement of others, it has a significant positive impact on everyone we come into contact with.

Over time, I have become very sensitive to these energy shifts. I can't remain in situations that are strongly negative anymore — the energy feels like it sucks the life out of me. You may know the situations I'm talking about; we might refer to these people as emotional vampires who seem to take from everyone they come into contact with.

There is a saying that we are a product of the five people we spend the most time with... Of course, once we understand the vibration of emotion, we can understand why people who spend a lot of time together would have to vibrate in a similar space most of the time. However, if someone new comes into that group, they can quickly bring down the whole group if they have a strong negative influence. Once we are aware of it, we can be much more proactive in ensuring the space around us is as positive as it can be, and we become very aware of when that energy shifts.

MANAGEMENT OF THE SYSTEM

This is a key component of ongoing management of our wellbeing. When we are more in touch with our own body and intuitively connected within our system, we can then recognise the shift and start to look for the catalyst for the change and take more immediate and affirmative action.

Then we have to add to that improved communication skills because the changes to our environment will be impacted by those around us. When we develop 'mastery' over our own system, we can be aware of how that impact occurred and we can communicate it to that person in a way which could easily resolve an issue before it develops into something much bigger.

We have to take ownership of our own thoughts, feeling and behaviours, and communicate that openly with those around us, so they may be able to assist us to resolve anything that feels negative. Of course, this is something that needs to be done with someone else who is hopefully just as self-aware — I'm hopeful that as more people read this book they will be able to assist others to see value in such an approach. It really is the only way for humanity to reach a point where we can improve our connections and grow and improve together.

Perhaps then we can positively influence the many things in our world that are in a downward spiral, hopefully before we manage to annihilate the human race... But it does feel like we are racing against time.

MODERNISATION

There are a number of issues that have affected humanity in the past 100 years — mainly as a direct result of industrialisation. Some of them have been great for humanity, and some have had a negative impact. Whichever way we look at it, we just need to recognise that it has had an impact.

This impact goes directly to the ability we have to resolve issues, and why some of the inventions of the 20th century may have assisted in the growth of economies, but I'm not 100% convinced it has been to the betterment of humanity.

Interestingly, there are a number of therapies now being utilised to assist us in the recovery of our mental health that are things we would have naturally experienced if we had not had significant growth in capitalism. Let's consider some of the issues; to do this I'm going to take us back 100 years to the period that was post the First World War, when the development of technology was really starting to ramp up. We developed new machinery, and the notion of capitalism really started to take hold in the western world. There was a lot of growth and development post-war; there were new cars, new pieces of machinery that assisted us in managing household tasks, and life became more 'modern'.

This was particularly so for women. There were major changes for women post-war. They were able to vote in most developed countries. They were able to wear shorter dresses; finally fashion was beginning to catch up with practicality. There was more opportunity for people to work hard and play hard. There was ready access to alcohol for the masses, and the divide between the 'landed gentry' and the common man started to break down.

But there were also challenges. The war had left some men quite damaged. What used to be referred to as 'shell shock' was known to affect many who had returned from the war, and their behaviour affected the loved ones they came home to. People made allowances for the behaviour, but not a lot was commonly known about mental health issues.

In fact, the field of psychology really only started around the turn of the century. A lot of interest in psychiatric study was coming out of Germany – from scholars such as Jung and Freud.[21] However, the 'father' of modern psychology is recognised as William James, who was an American, with his book *The Principles of Psychology*.

There have been major changes in our social fabric as a result of wars, each war leaving its unique mark on the psyche of the communities involved. However, it really hasn't been until the 1970s and the fallout of the Vietnam War that I think society has more fully understood how the impact of war then permeates through our societies. The full impact of these I may need to consider in my next book.

Time Pressures

As the world has adopted more and more mechanical, electrical and computerised systems that make certain processes more efficient, we have freed up that time and used it to work harder in other areas. Take the development of any machinery, be it domestic or industrial, and I can show you a piece of equipment which freed us up from one chore so we could work longer on a different task.

Is that such a big problem? Perhaps... Or perhaps not. But whichever way we look at it, we have freed ourselves from many domestic tasks to fill that time with tasks that contribute to further development – this is especially true in the industrialised world. By streamlining domestic tasks, we have made more time available for the further development of capitalism. It is also a self-propelling mechanism that industrialised nations have significantly supported, and it is fuelled by the desire to consume.

Now, I'm not about to launch into a speech on the evils of capitalism or the benefits of communism, because this isn't a political discussion. Besides which, it doesn't matter about our politics; the desire to consume drives economies.

What I want you to recognise is we have developed new things to free up our time, but all we did was fill that time with more things – more efficient and effective ways of doing things because we want to earn good money to enable us to afford to consume the things we desire. With the ever-increasing appetite of consumption, there can reach a point where the voracity cannot ever be satiated.

MODERN MOTHERHOOD

Technology was sold to us as a way to free up our time, but for many people it's had the opposite effect. It is the drive for more effective use of our time that has led to more problems in our society, because in the process we have also devalued the domestic tasks, especially the raising of our children.

In western societies, we give birth to our children and then we distance ourselves from them as the society does not place any value on our role as mothers. It is extremely rare in modern industrialised societies for a mother to be able to stay home with her child until they are ready to start school. There are women who don't want to stay home with their children because they feel it doesn't provide them with enough interaction or intellectual stimulation, but I would argue that this is because we don't afford them an effective community network that assists them to be valued and connected while they fulfil that role.

Don't misunderstand me — I am an absolute feminist and my role and my rights are equal to that of any male. However, I cannot refute the reality of my physiology. My body is capable of being impregnated and nurturing life — and without it the human race would not continue. If we stop having children then eventually we will become extinct.

I believe industrialised societies need to reframe their approach to the value of motherhood in our society, but generally I believe we need to value parenthood. It is in this area that I believe the Scandinavians really have a fantastic approach. They recognise supporting young mothers to raise healthy children is imperative to the prosperous future of their nations, so government support is provided to young families to ensure mothers are able to spend time nurturing their children and building strong communities.

THE IMPACT OF CHILDCARE

It has only been in the past 15 to 20 years that we started considering the impact of a range of care situations and how these might affect our children. Given what I have outlined earlier in this book, would spending time in childcare from the age of six weeks be more beneficial to the long-term mental health of a child? Or would the impact be negative? It's not hard to understand that the impact on our development would be negative, and emerging research appears to be supporting the fact that the mental health outcomes of children who spent their early years in the care of adults, other than their biological parents or grandparents, have significantly poorer mental health outcomes than those who don't.

So, the impact of time on our lives cannot be dismissed. We have saved a lot of time from the impact of modernisation to improve the speed and quality of our domestic tasks, however we haven't taken that time and improved the connection we have with our families. Instead, we have also reduced the time we spend with our children and other members of the family to drive ourselves to improve our financial outcomes, further driving our consumerism. It's a vicious cycle.

Environment

The other thing we have managed to do with our newfound technology is minimise our exposure to discomfort. We've all heard the phrase 'necessity is the mother of invention', but I would have to ask if, in fact, it is 'discomfort' that is the mother of invention.

There are many and varied treatments and recommendations for people to assist them to effectively manage, or improve, their mental health which are based on forcing ourself into discomfort. It seems the way humans have evolved over time means we have learned to create things that allow us to avoid extremes, thereby staying in a space in which we are not placed under any physiological stress. Although these things have helped us in many ways, it is clear it has been to our detriment.

I no longer have to get uncomfortable about anything. I move from my air-conditioned house, in my air-conditioned car to an air-conditioned office. I can buy prepared food everywhere I go – so I don't have to force myself to hunt or gather, unless it is at the organic farmers market on the weekend! If I don't 'feel' like doing anything – I don't have to force myself. I can lie on the couch, watch hours of Netflix and call Uber Eats when I get hungry. We live our lives on 'autopilot', with no insight into the source of the food we consume or how many chemicals or preservatives we are exposing our gut to, and we take multiple supplements to combat the lack of variety in our diet. Then we pass on these poor food habits to our children.

We have good community awareness of mental health issues, but often that facilitates dependency rather than supporting recovery.

Don't get me wrong – I have been that hard-working sole parent who bought prepared meals because I was busy, but I was aware that it really wasn't the best choice for my children. We have created a cycle of dependencies due to the increased pressure we feel to achieve more with less time, without a focus on the true values of our society – connecting with each other.

It is not surprising that we have developed a range of therapeutic interventions that actually seem to help us with our mental health by forcing our bodies into discomfort. From cold water therapies to pushing our physical bodies hard with intensive exercise, we are seeing improvements in mental health from engaging in activities that would have been part of our daily life 'pre-industrialisation'.

THE MEDITERRANEAN LIFESTYLE

There is a lot of discussion about the benefits of different ways of eating, and one of the consistent approaches that is considered beneficial for longevity is what's often known as 'the Mediterranean diet'. In essence, in that part of the world they eat more fish and fresh vegetables, low-fat dairy products, drink alcohol regularly but in moderation, and live a long time!

I am constantly amazed, however, that the other factors around the lifestyle of people who live in the Mediterranean are not taken into account – just what they eat. Yet, anyone who has visited countries that border the Mediterranean would know – the families all live together on family compounds, or are at least close by. There is intergenerational care of children, and family plots for growing vegetables and keeping a small number of livestock. Older people have purpose – they get up every morning and take their livestock to graze, collect eggs and ripe fruits and vegetables, and prepare meals. They congregate at the local cafes and drink coffee and chat – they connect. They connect with many and varied members of their communities and they feel a sense of belonging.

They also gossip, and there are many disagreements and unnecessary judgements made about people and between small villages, but their sense of family connection overrides everything. They know they belong — their daily lifestyle and connections demonstrate and reinforce their value to their community.

When I visited Greece recently, I witnessed firsthand how the village lifestyle can really help people to feel connected. It can feel suffocating to those of us from more Anglo–Saxon backgrounds, yet we can see how the role of each family member is valued and provides them with a sense of purpose. These cultures really do value parenting and grandparenting. The grandparents have an active role in the lives of their children and grandchildren. They farm family plots, raise chickens, milk sheep and barter the milk for cheese — then share these resources with the extended family. In this way, their lives have purpose until they pass on.

I will never forget watching my host's parents getting on with the daily tasks of life. They had moved into a smaller building on the family property, and the son had taken over the family home with his wife and children. Their daughter and her husband and children live around the corner. Every morning the patriarch of this family gets up and, with his wife and his oxygen bottle (he now has emphysema), they get in the old ute and take the sheep and goats down the hill to graze on the river flats. They collect from the food plot anything they might use that day. Then the grandmother starts preparing food while she helps out the grandchildren to get them ready for school. Their Mum has gone to work outside of the home, and their Dad does shift work. The grandfather walks down to the local café and plays cards with his mates until lunch, when he goes home and eats a meal with the family before having an afternoon nap. Then they collect the livestock, and grandmother milks the sheep and collects the milk to trade with the local cheese producer. The son helps out on the family plot, and the children will often spend time with their grandparents helping out. They all sit down after dinner with a night cap, and go to bed at a reasonable hour. Then they wake up to do it all again.

True, this is a level of subsistence living — hunter–gatherer style — and not really suited to our industrialised world. However, this is proving to the world how the ability to maintain connection and a level of purpose, coupled with daily exercise and wholesome organic foods, combine to produce robust and healthy human beings. Their life is more simplistic, and it wouldn't be for everyone. However, I don't believe we can ignore the fact that countries that value family connections and community values appear to be happier, healthier and live longer.

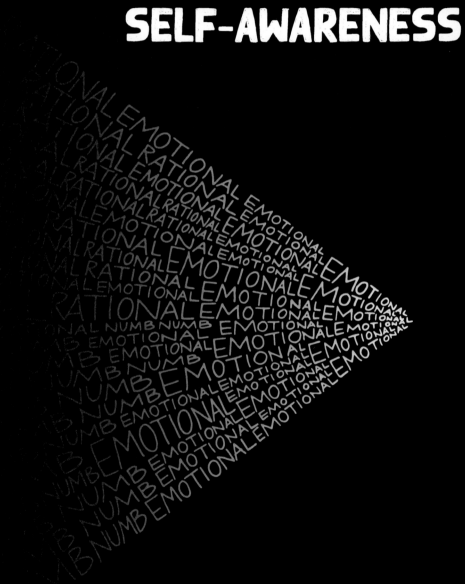

CHAPTER FIVE
SELF-AWARENESS

With True Self-Awareness
Comes Self-Acceptance
And A Good Sense
Of Self-Worth

As I outlined in chapter three, we need to understand ourselves and the true core of who we are as human beings, completely separate from how others perceive us. I referred to a guided meditation that provides us some insight into the central idea of who we are as a person, and clarity about the fact that the child within us is perfectly loveable and acceptable and deserving of love.

RECONNECTING TO SELF

The key to ongoing management of the system moving forward is in understanding that our four year old is the true basis of our ego, the core component to our personality, and we need to ensure this child is valued, heard and supported if we want to be able to live a truly happy and fulfilling life. Continuing to ignore or berate the child within us will result in an ongoing battle within that will never abate. Once we know that it is unnecessary, we just need to ensure we have a way to gain clarity and acceptance of our true self, and recognise when the child within us needs support and how to get it for them.

Clients of mine will often report they can develop awareness of their parts of self, but struggle to move between their aspects of self 'at will'. One of the fabulous things about engaging this technique is we can develop a way that stops all of the negative voices in our head for good! Yes — I am serious! When we have full acceptance of self, it gets very quiet in there!

I will never forget the moment of clarity I had about my own process in this. I have only reached this state of 'quiet nirvana' in my head in the past three years. I would say that over many years it has been getting quieter, but it wasn't until I had true acceptance between my child and protector parts and ongoing trust with my rational adult self that my internal chatter stopped. It took me a few weeks to realise it had happened, but the recognition was incredibly profound.

Our experiences shape us

I have done quite a lot of work on my own personal issues, including attachment issues. However, it wasn't until I did some therapy around my own inability to maintain a long-term, committed relationship that I started to really uncover how this process works. You see, I'm the youngest of five children, and I grew up in a sole-parent family. My older siblings have all been married for in excess of 30 years. I'm the only one of my siblings to have been married more than once, and I have had several longer term, committed relationships. I had resolved many of the challenges of my perception of myself and had really become accepting of myself, happy in my own skin, clear about who I am and what I can offer to the world. However, I was still struggling with intimate relationships.

I have had several co-dependent relationships over my life, not surprising really when we analyse how they form and what I need to feel valued in a relationship. However, I clearly felt I had resolved those issues several years ago after I came out of a relationship that I had developed with an old high school friend. I was very aware of the things I had done in ignoring the 'red flags' which had come up early in the relationship, and fully accepted my responsibility in allowing those red flags to be ignored. Consciously, I felt I was able to see what I had done and why, and I was okay with that. I also felt I would be prepared for any other opportunity in the future, to recognise I didn't need to compromise myself or my own values to support others. I honestly felt, for the first time in my life, that I was okay just as I was, and that if someone else couldn't see that, due to their own issues, it was not my responsibility to fix that for them. I felt truly liberated.

I then had a period of 'dating' — I'm going to be honest and say this was the first period of real dating I had ever done, for in truth I was a serial monogamist. I had moved from one long-term relationship to another, making constant allowances for the men I was in a relationship with. I obtained a certain sense of my own value from being able to help others with their problems. This natural tendency for self-sacrifice is probably what drove me to psychology in the first instance, but it was really very damaging for me and my personal relationships.

So, I actually revelled in this 'dating' period in my life, and see it as a marker of my true liberation from co-dependency. I am proud of the fact I had a period of time where I had several connections that lasted no more than one month, as it takes about three weeks for the first 'red flag' to start, and if we are being true to ourself, we don't ignore that. If we choose to ignore it the first time, it will raise its head again around six weeks, and again at three months. When we are fully accepting of ourself, we do not ignore these 'red flags' in the belief that we can help resolve the problem for the other person, or worse, with the belief that we can change someone else.

When I finally did enter into another long-term relationship, I honestly felt it was the best one of my life. I felt supported and accepted. We had shared values and common goals. We had effective and open communication and mutual respect. There was honesty – or so I thought. At least, I was being honest.

That relationship lasted a year, and ended abruptly. I really struggled with that. Firstly, I had always been the one who ended my relationships. For the first time in my life, someone else was rejecting me – openly. Secondly, I struggled with this because we had never had any problems, or at least I wasn't aware of any. Therein lay the issue... I was operating in the relationship with honesty and transparency. I was treating him the way I wanted to be treated and it was working extremely well. I assumed that the other person was doing the same. Unfortunately, he wasn't.

It took me quite a long time to get over the ending of this relationship, mainly because I couldn't understand the problem and he wouldn't be honest with me about it. As it turned out, he was very good at keeping his views to himself, and only allowing them to be expressed under extreme pressure, at which point a volcano would erupt. He had learned to 'control' his anger, but ultimately he knew that if I saw it for what it truly was I wouldn't want to be around it. He had struggled to control it his whole life, and had deluded himself into believing it was resolved because he was able to control it better. In reality, he had just learned to suppress it and avoid situations he knew would trigger it — that's not resolving the underlying issue, it's trying to control the surface to make it appear as if things are calm, despite the constant rumbling of the volcano.

HOW OUR PHYSIOLOGICAL ENVIRONMENT IMPACTS OUR CELLULAR FUNCTIONING

When I was finally able to get to the bottom of the issue, I was then able to let go. I had to accept that he wasn't able to be honest with himself, let alone allow me into his head to try to assist him to resolve the problem. This is where I believe I was truly able to liberate myself. I had come a long way to understanding and accepting myself as a person, recognising my imperfections and challenges, but being able to love myself regardless. He had come a long way within himself, but he still wasn't able to face the reality of his own issues. However, I wasn't able to help him with that; he had to come to a place where he could see that for himself.

I went to see my supervisor (what psychologists term their own therapists), and I engaged in some therapy around this issue I had with relationships and the reality that this issue linked all the way back to my experience as a baby in utero. I would ask the sceptic in you to just stay with me on this for a short while, as it is critical to understanding how the physiological environment we are in impacts our cellular functioning in ways we do not consciously recognise.

During this therapy session, I was able to see that in all of my previous relationships I was chasing the acceptance of my father. The personality similarities were clear to me, but after my high school connection I was able to put that clearly behind me and I sought a different kind of relationship. With this most recent relationship, I was chasing the validation of my mother. For many and varied reasons — that I won't go into here out of respect for my relationship with my Mum — I recognised I had clearly sought a different kind of relationship to help me resolve my disconnect from my mother.

Surprisingly, in this therapy session I became aware I had been conceived into a womb that did not want me. I need to reinforce the fact that this wasn't my mother's fault, and I don't blame her at all for any of this. However, the reality of my conception was I had not been planned. I think it would also be fair to say that my parents' relationship was already under strain. They had four children already, ranging in age from seven to three; the surprise of another mouth to feed would have made things challenging for any young family. The recognition of the subconscious experience of not being wanted went to the fabric of my cells and laid the blueprint for the sense of needing to 'prove' my value to be able to obtain a secure attachment and survive.

This experience was later reinforced when my father finally left us when I was 15 months old. My mother never blamed me, but I feel like she wondered whether or not he would have stayed if I hadn't been born.

If you ask her now, she would say clearly that our lives were greatly improved without his involvement, but it was tough. Mum really struggled financially for the first year, before someone told her she was able to obtain some government support to assist her to raise us. But it was difficult... I know she struggled. I'm sure she was depressed for a while, and I was the only one with her, day in and day out, as all the older kids were at school by this stage.

Even at only 15 months, there was an underlying fear I experienced from the loss of both of my parents — my father physically and my mother emotionally. It wasn't their fault; they didn't even understand the impact it would have on how I would perceive myself. But I was doing everything I could to ensure that I didn't lose the one person who was still physically present. Is it any surprise I felt I needed to help her? Even though I was only a baby, my need to maintain connection was activated.

As my mother tells it, I was the one thing that used to bring them all out of the sadness. I was a happy baby, and gave all of them a welcome distraction from their fears and the challenges that lay ahead for the next 12 months. However, during the day they were at school, and it was just me alone with my depressed Mum. Research shows that depressed mothers create emotional instability in their babies because they are emotionally disconnected. To add to her depression, my father had left her with no top teeth. You see, each successive pregnancy had leeched the calcium from her teeth, and during her pregnancy with me they removed all of her top teeth. Can you imagine what that fear and pain must have done to me in utero?

Mum had remained without any top teeth for 18 months. She was struggling to feed us, let alone being able to afford to buy herself a new set of false teeth. My father's parting gift to her was to buy her a new set of teeth — in the hope she would get a better paying job and relieve him of the burden of having to support us.

He was a selfish man.

The important thing to understand is there were many and varied reasons my experience of abandonment was very different to that of my siblings. We were all affected by our parents' divorce, in many different ways. There are many reasons we are all grateful he left, especially because I think it afforded us an opportunity to gain strength that we may not have otherwise found if our mother had not eventually found her own sense of self-worth. She found it within herself, but she would never again allow a man to determine her value. My mother remains a single, independent woman to this day — almost 50 years later.

But that is another story.

The basis of our issues are usually set in childhood

It is important we understand how our experiences shape us. Modern psychology will often focus on addressing the issues that are 'current', but the basis of our issues are usually set in childhood. We know adverse childhood experiences impact our health, and my childhood certainly was not free from adversity. However, I find the focus of the ACEs questionnaire is on extreme trauma and abandonment; it isn't geared to pick up many of the circumstances like I have just shared with you. Yet, it is clear my emotional challenges around forming intimate relationships have been significantly impacted by the reality of my very early life.

I have outlined my awareness of the challenges that have developed from my very early childhood, yet I do not have many specific memories from my early years. It's because we don't recall this information that we believe it doesn't impact us, yet it clearly changes the way our cells respond to our emotional experiences. However, it is not until the age of four that we become consciously aware of our sense of ourselves as 'separate'. As outlined earlier, this is when we start to accept the responsibility of managing our feelings and being held to account for our behaviour. This is the basis of our true self, and we need to be able to provide ourselves with the love and acceptance we desperately craved from others, but for varying reasons we were unable to experience.

It is my sincerest wish that you are able to connect with your inner child and truly be able to see how perfect they are. When we are able to do this, the world becomes a much easier place to navigate, as we are not trying to navigate it in avoidance, running from our fear of abandonment.

RECOVERY RATHER THAN SURVIVAL

At the very beginning of this book I outlined why it's important to understand that we don't want to be 'survivors' of our life experiences, rather we choose to be persistent 'recoverers'.

What I am hoping we take from this book is an understanding of how our traumatic experiences have affected our development. How we learn behaviours and our standard responses to our day-to-day experiences have a strong link to all of the other traumatic experiences we have had that made us feel the same way. In trauma therapy we often refer to our 'triggers', the experiences we have that activate a similar feeling to what we have had previously, usually activating either one of our two primary negative emotions – fear or shame. As a result, we 'react' to the current situation as if it was the same as the original experience, even though we have no conscious connection between the two.

As such, we tend to view ourselves as 'overreacting' to something, but we often don't have any awareness of this until after the fact, and only then if we make a conscious decision to try to understand our behaviour. This is where our ability to build our self-awareness is extremely important; without it we cannot recover.

SELF-AWARENESS NOT SELF-INVOLVEMENT

A lot of psychological interventions are designed to improve our self-awareness. Like anything, we can have 'too much' of a good thing. Some people take the concept of self-awareness to a whole new level – over-thinking every action they take or word they say. At this point we tip over the edge of awareness into paranoia.

Being self-aware is a difficult skill to master. There are many who would consider themselves to be self-aware, but they think that means their needs can be expressed to everyone around them. This is really self-involvement. Their awareness of what they want then becomes everyone else's problem to deliver. These people often get frustrated that they can't get what they want because other people don't give it to them.

If they were truly self-aware, they would recognise they need to work out how to meet that need for themselves, and understand that when others don't meet it for them they will feel understandably sad and hurt, but the problem is still theirs to resolve.

Remember what I said about needing to be unconditionally loved? We often look to others to validate us in many and varied ways and prove to us that we are loveable. However, the truly self-aware know they are loveable. They love themselves enough to ask those who care about them to help them, and give them certain considerations to support their relationship growth, but ultimately, they have enough self-worth to recognise the emotional needs they have and seek to find ways to fill them. With true self-awareness comes self-acceptance and a good sense of self-worth.

We have to resolve our traumatic injuries to be able to reach the point where we can have a good sense of self-acceptance and recognition of our self-worth. To understand what issues we need to resolve, we need to work on becoming more self-aware.

This is where psychological therapies can help us to explore the challenges we have overcome in our life. Unfortunately, for most of us, our perception of overcoming an issue is usually indicative of the ability to repress the feelings associated with the experience. We just decide not to think about it, push the feelings away or avoid the source of the pain. As we can see, none of those words indicate an issue has been resolved, rather we just try to ignore it.

Overcoming ego

There are many who would also believe they have a great sense of their self-worth, but these people have often built their self-worth on 'what' they do, rather than 'who' they are.

This is extremely common in western societies, and growing in eastern societies. When you consider what I have outlined about how our sense of ourselves is formed through our childhood, when we are encouraged to externalise our feelings and seek validation from external sources about our worth, is it any surprise that many of us think our sense of self is about our work? We have made our 'work' to be representative of our purpose — yet these are entirely unrelated.

If it's not work, we can often validate ourselves by other achievements — sporting or academic achievements. These days we see many young people validate themselves by how many Instagram followers they have, or the number of Facebook friends they have. There is a major problem with this approach, as it is the ultimate externalisation of our perception of ourselves. It's based on what other people, most of whom are complete strangers, think of our image or our experiences.

This is why many young people experience challenges with their mental health, because at the time of their life when they are developmentally programmed to establish connections with their peers, they believe social media platforms represent the reality of those connections.

When I was in high school, I only needed to concern myself with the bullies on the school bus or the rumours going around my year group about me — all still traumatic experiences in and of themselves. However, the bullies could not anonymously attack me, or question my actions or tarnish my reputation in a public forum that was theoretically able to be viewed by the whole planet.

We now have a whole generation of young adults who were raised in an age of open access to all sorts of information thanks to the development of technology. They have no concept of the world before the internet and mobile phones.

Now, I love technology and embrace it, however I am also aware that when it is not managed well, it can lead to significant problems. I see it a lot when I'm working with children — they have no concept of life without personal devices. Their attention spans are reducing, and their ability to retain information is not great. After all, they don't need to retain information — they have all the information in the world available at their fingertips.

I'm not a naysayer, I'm a realist. We can't take away the technology, but we can try to raise awareness about balancing its use with other pursuits — like making billycarts and baking cakes. Unfortunately, as parents our lives have become busier, and as a result we don't have a lot of time with our kids to do these types of activities.

The challenge for us as a community is we need to be able to raise awareness and try to put in place some mechanisms which will support our young people to reconnect with themselves. We can do this by validating the expression of emotion in our children, rather than just trying to dominate our perspective over the top of theirs.

RECOVERY REQUIRES BALANCE

Our approach needs balance though, as most processes that seek to validate a particular position often end up creating an extreme reaction to the newly validated phenomenon.

Let me give you some examples. You will recall prior to the 1980s, no one really talked about child abuse; in fact, verbal and physical abuse was considered normal 'parenting'. Sexual abuse was never talked about, and children who did speak up about it were often called liars.

In the past few years, we have come to understand how wide-spread the problem really is and how it has permeated through many of our community settings, like churches and sporting groups. So, as parents, we've limited our children's exposure to this threat by minimising their interactions with the outside world.

Yes, we are protecting them, but we are also not helping them to learn how to problem solve their way through difficulties — in many cases we have wrapped them in cotton wool and given them the idea that the whole world is a dangerous place. As a result, they don't develop the skills to know how to cope with some of life's challenges.

Another example is bullying and harassment in the workplace. Twenty years ago, this kind of behaviour was just accepted as part of an organisation's culture. However, as our awareness has grown as to what bullying and harassment is, people start to see it every-where. It's become so commonplace that any person expressing a strong opinion can now be accused of bullying.

It's normal for us to move from one extreme position to another one; it is how our brain assists us to overcome our previous bias. I mentioned earlier about how our brain supports us to accept a new way of thinking or viewing the world, by making us more supportive of it than if we had just accepted it in the first place. We then become fierce advocates of the new way as a mechanism to overcome how negatively we viewed it in the first instance.

Think about how a 'reformed smoker' approaches people who smoke. Or how someone who has become a vegetarian might approach their friends who still eat meat. To validate our decision to do something differently, we can often judge those who are still doing things the old way much more harshly than if we were always accepting of the new position.

When we view this at the community level, it manifests in extremism. At a global level, it starts wars.

Those who are truly self-aware tend to be more balanced in their approach towards others, accepting that they have a right to live however they want and not feel the pressure of being judged by others. To become self-aware, we may need to do quite a bit of therapy work and be able to connect within ourself, emotionally and physically.

CHAPTER SIX
EMPOWERMENT

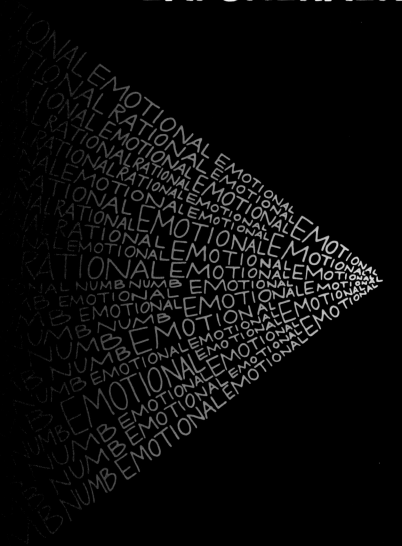

The Key To Recovery
Rests In Our Ability
To Feel A Sense Of Purpose
After The Experience

Once we understand that trauma is at the basis of all of our negative emotional experience and it causes us to have physical issues in addition to psychological ones, we need a process to follow to enable us to recover.

Negative emotion causes cellular changes in our body, which is why over the course of time, our physical bodies often deteriorate. Our immune systems change, and we often just put that down to ageing. However, we are learning more through neuroscience research every day about how our brains are capable of change, and neuroplasticity tells us we can change anything and everything about ourselves.

I have outlined in the previous chapter the need to be self-aware. Without being able to get in touch with our own thoughts, feelings and behaviours, we are unable to change anything. The process of recovery cannot happen without first having a clear purpose for our experiences and our lives. Once we're clear on our purpose, which affords us a sense of value, we then need to build our self-awareness. We need to do that at an emotional level, but we also need to do that from a physical perspective. I want to outline a variety of techniques and systems you might like to try to support you with recovery.

RECOVERY

In the preface of this book I talked about purpose and how the ability to recover is dependent on it.

When we understand that our traumatic experiences over time impact our ability to feel like we have a purpose, it's easier to understand why some people find a recovery process more difficult than others.

The impact from any traumatic experience is directly related to our sense of responsibility in the experience, our lack of control or power in the face of the experience, and our ability to attribute meaning to why we had the experience.

In terms of negative experiences that cause bigger problems in the long term, the real issue comes down to whether or not we blame ourself, or something or someone else. Is it me (internal) as opposed to that or them (external)? Experiences we feel responsible for have a much more significant impact than experiences we know are not our fault — even when the outcome could be far worse.

COMMUNITY TRAUMA

As I have written this book, Australia was first affected by a significant bushfire crisis. The impact was unprecedented, and we thought that 2020 could not have had a worse start — until the coronavirus. In fact, the publication of this book was directly impacted by a pandemic — unlike anything the world has seen before.

Sure — we have had a variety of pandemics in our human history, but we haven't been able to see the actual enormity of the death and destruction from our own living rooms. As I write, there is civil unrest that is impacting the United States and there are demonstrations going on all around the world.

What causes all of this unrest? I have written about the impact of change in varying forums in the past, but there is nothing like what we are seeing right now — and many people may be wondering 'why now'?

There is a phenomenon that occurs when people are forced to make change. When COVID-19 first became an issue in early 2020, Australia was still reeling from a bushfire crisis and the real threat of coronavirus was not widely felt in Australia. It was March before the spread and the true contagious nature of the virus was clearly understood and it was mid-March before our government, along with many other countries around the world, decided to take a very strong stand about the need to protect its citizens from the threat.

I am very aware that we live in 'The Lucky Country'. We are truly blessed. We live in a democratic, economically stable, socialist society and, as such, our government had the means and the controls to be able to place the country into 'hibernation'. I have many friends and colleagues who live in other parts of the world, and it has been amazing to see the many and varied ways that governments all around the world have responded to this crisis.

From the incredible leadership of New Zealand and Greece to the unbelievable arrogance of Brazil – we have seen incredible stories of camaraderie and care, as well as unbelievable stories of stupidity and greed.

If I look back to what I first outlined in chapter two about Gaia Theory and the need for mother earth to rebalance an over-populated planet when the planet becomes imbalanced – perhaps that is one explanation for a situation like coronavirus. One thing is for sure, the virus impacts the weak and frail most significantly and yet children appear to be relatively unaffected (although I am aware that there is a slight variation that appears to be affecting children who potentially have less robust immune systems).

It is not my intention to get into a debate about the purpose of a pandemic, except to say that it is an incredible 'leveller' of our society. It has been incredibly difficult, but it has also brought with it some amazing opportunities and given us the chance to refocus on what is truly important – our health and our families.

One of the things that it has done is make people stop and focus on their home lives. Many parents had to take the time to educate their children at home and take the time to break up their day by taking their children outside and interacting with them in different ways. One of the most incredible things that happened is that people started spending more time doing physical activities in their family units – in our local area there was an 800% increase in bicycle path usage in the month of April!

We've seen really interesting things happen in addition to increased bicycle usage; we have cooked at home more and taken the time to prepare meals together. Working online for most people means that they are not wanting to have more screen time in the evenings – many families have returned to playing board games and reading books – real paper books, not ebooks. Audiobooks also saw an increase as people didn't want to over-use their eyes any further.

I noticed it – I was able to move immediately to working online with clients – but I was getting headaches at the end of each day and I had to go and get new glasses that are especially for screen usage. In many ways, our ability to transition to online is great for maintaining social connection and interaction in a 'safe' way – but as most of us were working online, we ended up feeling like we didn't want to interact via screen anymore.

I really noticed the usual 'adaption' timeframes when everyone was reporting how low they were feeling – three weeks, six weeks, and now we are approaching three months as I write this, and many people are feeling a bit low and lethargic. These are the standard timeframes of human adaption – it is the same as when we experience any change in our environment that is not of our own choice.

You will notice this phenomenon if you have ever travelled overseas for an extended period, or if you have ever moved a long way away from your hometown. We have these periods of adaption as our brain is programmed to identify and address the 'difference'.

The power of three is not just a mathematical phenomenon – it's how our brains like to process information according to psychological theory. Our brain needs certainty to settle our anxiety. At this time our brain is screaming for us to find a solution to the things that are outside of our control – so that we can feel more comfortable in it.

Many people would be aware of the power of three in our lives – it is a commonly known principle. Three weeks to change a habit – three weeks to adapt. Our brain can engage in something 'novel' for about three weeks before there is a push back. To begin with it's unfamiliar and interesting, but after about three weeks our brain wants to go back to 'normal'. You see, our body and brain likes homeostasis − we like things to be familiar and remain the same. Novelty is interesting for a period of time and, depending on our personality, some of us are more open to novelty than others. Regardless, the cycle of three is one that can be observed.

So, after three weeks, we see our first period of adaption. Three weeks, six weeks, three months, six months... After the six-month mark, we have adjusted to our new lifestyle so much that we could essentially live like this forever. However, when things are imposed on us, this same timeframe phenomena also comes into play − but it presents quite differently. The three-week mark is the first point where our brain says, 'Enough! − I don't like this anymore'. Then again at six weeks − and after that each stage doubles, three months, six months, one year and two years. Each cycle raises a grief cycle as we try to adapt to the different experiences.

As with the stages of grief we go through a variety of feelings: Denial − 'It's just a flu − we'll be fine!' Anger − 'You can't stop my civil liberties... I have a right to go wherever I want!' Bargaining − 'I wonder if I can just go to one friend's house?' Depression − 'I really don't want to live like this − I hate it!' Acceptance − 'Actually! I think I could work from home forever!'

With coronavirus it is the uncertainty that created bigger issues as it meant that most of us were in limbo for extensive periods of time, unable to make big decisions. As the fear settled around our health, it began to rise about our financial future. We need to make some 'interim' decisions on how we will cope, so that we can move forward. It's the uncertainty that creates more difficulties.

We need to recognise that each trip to the supermarket makes us feel unsafe due to COVID-19 and we have all been vibrating in fear. We feel it. Things are starting to settle down for many of us as the routines have started to kick back in. However, if we haven't set any routines, it will create more challenges.

As we adapt to any change, we adapt the way that we approach things and it takes quite a while to change back. In reality, the life of a pandemic is three to five years, and our need to remain socially distant and mindful of hygiene will remain with us for many years to come. The fabric of our society has changed forever, and it won't ever go back to the way that it was. It brings with it opportunities and difficulties — we just need to work out how to overcome the difficulties to ensure we can embrace the opportunities.

One of the unique things about traumatic experience that is experienced by whole communities, rather than just as individuals, is that it doesn't feel quite so personal. We still have to process the grief and work through our individual losses, but the impact is spread across the community as our grief is shared.

What we need to be mindful of is the burden of compounding trauma, such as the potential for our bushfire-affected communities to be more significantly affected by COVID-19 and the resulting economic downturn, than their fellow Australians. It is true that there is a mediating effect from the experience being community wide, but when there is no time to recover before another negative experience comes along, the burden on these communities is compounded and significant.

In similar ways to frontline workers, the impact of recurrent trauma results in the physical body feeling inadequately prepared to respond. What is important is rather than accepting that this is just 'par for the course', an unintended consequence that just has to be dealt with, that we utilise this opportunity to provide widespread psychoeducation to these communities about their experiences, normalising them and providing insight into how they may be able to move forward and recover.

Purpose

The key to recovery rests in our ability to feel a sense a purpose after the experience. It doesn't matter what the traumatic experience is — workplace injury, child abuse, car accident, bushfire or pandemic... The key to recovery is in finding some reasonable position either for 'why' it happened or 'how' it can be used to help ourself or others in the future.

When we look at traumatic experiences it can be difficult to find a position for 'why' it happened, but it can be beneficial to feel we might be able to prevent the same thing happening to others in the future. In this way, the experience finds a purpose. A big part to being able to process this notion is to be able to work through the event to recognise what we are really responsible for and what we are not.

Traumatic experiences from childhood are often linked to irrational beliefs regarding responsibility for the experience. Developmentally our brains are still maturing and in childhood our prefontal cortex, which is responsible for higher order thinking, planning and judgement, is immature and that is why we have concrete, black or white thinking. If we have these experiences in childhood and they are not resolved, we will feel more responsible for traumatic experiences in adulthood. In this way, many people will find that they seem to have a lot of traumatic experiences in comparison to their friends or colleagues. However, it is often the perception of responsibility that results in us feeling situations that happen in our life are our fault — whether they rationally are or not.

In the same way, when trauma impacts a community, we often see people banding together to create change — rebuild or change laws. If we observe the civil unrest we are seeing in societies around the world at the moment, we are observing a social psychological phenomenon around group activation and change that hasn't been observed around the world since the 1960s. The reason for this is that people are becoming uncomfortable — it is in discomfort that things become unstable and there is more likely social agitation and unrest. It is much easier to create major change when things are unstable as our brains crave stability and certainty — homeostasis.

When things become unstable for the whole community it is much easier for people to behave in ways that they wouldn't if life was 'business as usual'. There is a sense that 'I have nothing to lose — but potentially a lot to gain' when things in our community are unstable. I won't bore you with all of the theories around social change and group theories, but suffice to say that what we are observing is quite normal and expected given the instability around the world.

We need to recognise that as human beings we are ultimately social beings who operate as individuals within varying units — families, communities and societies. We have to balance the needs of the individual with the needs of the varying groups to which that individual belongs and it is often a very delicate balance. At it's very core, if we all take ownership of resolving the traumatic injury to ourselves as individuals and we increase our awareness of how that impacts our interpersonal relationships, we will improve the outcomes for ourselves and *all* of society.

LIVING WITHOUT JUDGEMENT

When we look at where disagreements manifest in this world, there is always judgement involved. The unrest that is publicised by news services across the globe is always due to the differences between groups, or the individuals who belong to particular groups, and the disagreement that develops when they hold different perspectives about life.

In psychology we talk about group dynamics — the sense of belonging that we get from feeling that we belong to a particular group. These groups can range from families, to schools and universities, through to community groups that come together for a shared purpose. Conflict develops where one group judges another group and believes that they are better than them.

At the most basic level, it happens between sporting groups. We play with or support a team, and they compete against another group to show who is better at a particular activity. This competition is often seen as a leisure activity, used to demonstrate the effectiveness of one group's skills in a game when directly compared to another group's skills. However, there is a whole lot of social interaction going on around these types of activities and they strongly reflect human behaviour in other areas of life.

You know when people talk about football, how some people openly admit that their dedication to it is 'like a religion'? It's absolutely true. This helps us to understand how some sporting events, such as football matches, have ended in riots and other hugely negative outcomes. We can extend the analogy to the whole of society, for a wide variety of different groups, but in the end, the contention can only develop through judgement.

If there is one thing I wish for in this world, it would be that we all seek to live our lives minimising judgement. If we did this across the globe — then there would truly be world peace.

I have even written about this in my earlier books. In my contribution to *Better Business, Better Life, Better World* (see Appendix) I talk about the fact that if I could change one thing in this world it would be to eliminate unnecessary judgement.

In *Define Your Inner Diva* I talk about the need to minimise judgement. I have outlined in this book more about my early experience with organised religion and why I choose not to be involved with it.

As a society we have been taught our whole lives to disconnect from our bodies, not to feel things and not to react to things. Some of us have become so good at this that we believe that we don't get stressed or bothered by anything, yet we have persistent gut issues or find ourselves numbing ourselves to our emotions by drinking or over eating.

Gaining better awareness of our mind is actually the combination of our thoughts and our physical feelings. When we process negative emotional experiences they always have related physical sensations, so we need to be able to get in touch with our physical feelings, to develop embodied self-awareness.

CONNECTING TO OUR BODIES

'If every eight year old in the world is taught meditation, we will eliminate violence from the world within one generation.'

The Dalai Lama made this statement in 2012. There were many who questioned the wisdom of oversimplifying such a significant issue as violence; which has plagued humanity for all of our years. But I understand what he was trying to get at.

If you think about how I described that as a society we raise our children to externalise their thoughts and feelings and look to others to validate them, we can understand what the Dalai Lama is really trying to convey. He is saying we need to teach our children to get in touch with their physical body and observe themselves.

Let's look at some ways we can all connect to our bodies.

MENTAL EXERCISES

Meditation

According to the Buddhist Centre, meditation techniques encourage and develop clarity, concentration, emotional positivity and insight to the true nature of things.[22]

Through meditation we learn the patterns and habits of our mind, and it assists people to cultivate new, more positive ways of being. It is of no great surprise then that elements of meditation practices have been intertwined with psychology principles and promoted to the world as 'mindfulness' (see below).

It really doesn't matter what form of meditation we adopt, there is ample evidence people feel their mental health improves with meditation. Most people find that maintaining their mental state is easier if they practise mindfulness, or adopt standardised breathing techniques.

Mindfulness

Mindfulness is often used as a therapeutic technique. In essence, it is conscious awareness that is achieved by focusing on the present moment, while calmly acknowledging and accepting any thoughts, feelings or body sensations that come up. It is often combined with other psychological therapies to enhance outcomes. It improves our self-awareness.

My perspective on recovery is that when we have been able to eliminate the impact of our past experiences on our life, and we have resolved any fears we have of the future, then we can approach each day mindfully.

However, anyone who has tried this will know that it's very difficult to continue to stay focused on the present if our day-to-day existence is activating fear and shame. It is a great practice to learn, but if the underlying issues are still there then mindfulness can be seen as just another way of avoiding the feelings.

Big Mind, Big Heart

I came across this book about ten years ago. Like many of the works I have come across over my life, the way *Big Mind Big Heart* describes our different aspects of self really aligned with my perspectives. In his book, *Zen Master* Dennis Genpo Merzel employs a Jungian voice dialogue technique that enables people to understand their system in a way that seems manageable. Utilising his approach enabled me to become aware of my direct connection to all of humanity. It was an incredibly simple process to activate my 'big mind–big heart' – awareness and to tap into the unconditional compassion that we all can experience.

MIND–BODY EXERCISES

There has been great focus on the ability to use the mind to control the body, but also more recently on the ability to use specific movements in the body to control the mind.

Mind–body exercises may improve body function and overall health as they are shown to activate varying components of our nervous system, affecting our endocrine and immune systems. Today we are much more aware of how much our breathing affects us physically and mentally. Qigong, Tai Chi and Yoga are considered the most popular mind–body exercises, ranked as the top three most common complementary health approaches.[23]

Breath work

Breath work is a method of breath control that is meant to give rise to altered states of consciousness and to have an effect on physical and mental wellbeing.[24]

In a similar way to the rise of mindfulness in therapeutic work, there are many proponents of the value of controlled breathing techniques. As we are much more aware of the impact breathing has on our nervous system, we can also be aware of how our nervous system impacts our breathing. Anyone who has experienced a panic attack will be acutely aware of the impact it has on our bodies' usual approach to drawing breath.

Qigong and Tai Chi

Qigong is an ancient Chinese system of body postures and move-ment with coordinated breathing techniques and meditation. Qigong has roots in Chinese medicine, philosophy and martial arts.[25]

Tai Chi is considered more like a martial art or specific type of movement meditation with controlled breath work.[23] Interestingly, Qigong and Tai Chi together mirror many of the practices and philosophies of the Indian counterpart, yoga. Qigong practices include moving and still meditation, massage, chanting, sound med-itation and non-contact treatments, performed in a broad array of body postures.

Yoga

Yoga involves a combination of muscular activity and an internally directed mindful focus on awareness of the self, the breath and energy. Yoga integrates an individual's' physical, mental and spiritual components to improve physical and mental health, particularly stress-related illnesses.[26] Yoga incorporates additional elements that help maintain a connection to community and a sense of moral obli-gation to others, while maintaining the duality of the external and the internal.

There are many different traditions in yoga. Without focusing on the religious elements, the main purpose of applying yogic prin-ciples to our life centres around the connection to our body. The practice of yoga involves living by the seven spiritual laws of yoga, outlined over 5000 years of Vedic wisdom.

When I first started regularly engaging in yoga classes, my teacher was trained in the Satyananda tradition. According to that tradition, yoga is: a union between the individual and the cosmic self; a universal science of self-discovery, which evolved from the lifestyle and practices of the ancient seers; a comprehensive and practical system of transforming the human personality, which leads to balanced development of physical health, mental harmony and spiritual upliftment; a lifestyle that can change the quality of body and mind, allowing us to understand and fulfil our true potential; a positive way to enhance our creativity and expression in life through the unfolding of deeper dimensions of consciousness; a system that has a unique and universal appeal and may be practised by people from all walks of life, on all continents and of all religions; a practical philosophy which can create better human conditions and situations around the globe; the nature of all yogic practices is psycho-physiological — designed to improve mental control over our physical beings by raising the awareness and conscious connection to our bodies. Yoga practices include:

- Yama and Niyama (moral compass)

- Asana (steady postures)

- Pranayama (controlled breathing)

- Mudras and Bandhas (holds that activate the autonomic nervous system)

- Shat Kriya (cleansing processes)

- Dhyana (meditation)[27]

Modern life has shown us yoga in many forms in our society, most of them about the area of yoga referred to as the 'Asanas' — the physical postures. When we see all of the practices outlined as they are above, we can see how several practices within yoga have been separated as standalone approaches to many and varied issues in society.

In essence, yoga encompasses many processes that facilitate a connection to our bodies, allowing us to have some embodied self-awareness, an idea that is beginning to emerge as essential to our ability to resolve our physiological and psychological challenges.[9] Many yoga practices have been merged with psychology due to the growing awareness of the neurobiological connection between our mind and our body, strengthening our ability to allow one to control the other.

The thing I most like about yoga is that it is completely open to whatever beliefs we choose to have. Essentially, the seven laws of yoga encourage us to see ourselves as energy beings who are connected to all consciousness. As such, we are encouraged to accept the pure potential of our life, ensure that we give and receive, recognise the cause and effect of our actions (Karma), know that we can get what we want with the least effort, actively set our intentions to achieve our desires, and know the benefits of relinquishing control and the importance of fulfilling our life purpose.

INTEGRATIVE THERAPIES

Over the past 20 years there has been a variety of complementary or integrative therapies that are proving to have a positive impact on our psychological functioning. There are a range of emerging ideas people are adopting to manage our mental health and improve our physical health.[28]

When we consider the focus of many of these therapies, it's clear they are filling the gap in our physiological experiences that we no longer have to face due to the modern way of living, post industrialisation. Recall what I outlined about the fact that we no longer have to force ourselves to feel uncomfortable; well, as you can see, most of these emerging approaches are pushing our physical bodies to some level of extreme.

It doesn't really surprise me that pushing our physical body to extremes would be having an impact on our varying systems. There are a number of different examples of how our body responds to extreme pressure in varying forms – including the impacts from deprivation of one source or another, and even to the benefits of intermittent pressure. These approaches more recently have shown to have positive impacts on our body in everything from weight loss to improving muscle mass and fitness.

It's really interesting to observe how we are evolving as human beings when many of the things we normally have done over thousands of years in adapting to our environment are then overlaid with our industrialised world. In essence, we no longer have to adapt, so do we then stop evolving?

The health profession is really starting to come to life around the linkages between our physical health and our mental health, and that the key to recovery is to treat holistically. The advancement of our understanding of psycho–neuro–immunology has led to the establishment of organisations such as Integrative Medicine for Mental Health.

As such, I have outlined below some of the different therapies which are starting to be adopted in integrative approaches, but this is by no means comprehensive. There are new approaches being developed all the time. What is important here is that I believe you should adopt an approach that works for you, and it can be beneficial to engage in a few different therapies at the same time.

Light exposure

Light therapy was originally developed to treat seasonal affective disorder (SAD), a lowering of mood that occurs seasonally, usually with the onset of cooler weather. Exposure to artificial light is thought to affect brain chemicals linked to mood and sleep, and may also help with other mental health issues and sleep disorders. There are a variety of light therapy devices on the market, and there is quite a lot of research about the benefits of light therapy.

While I was in Europe a few years ago I was looking for a light therapy device. They are more commonly used in countries further away from the equator, as those countries have longer periods of darkness during winter, so there is greater awareness in those communities about the impact of light on mood. It was here that I discovered Valkee, now marketed as 'HumanCharger'.[29]

Researchers at the University of Oulu, Finland, discovered that in addition to our eyes, areas of the human brain are also sensitive to light. This sensitivity is due to the photoreceptor proteins in the brain, which are similar to those found in the eyes. Thinking outside the box, they found that brain areas can be reached by light through the ear canals, ear tissue and the skull — apparently the skulls of mammals let light pass through naturally. In ordinary daylight and daytime conditions, our brain is constantly being exposed to light, through our eyes and our skull.

In addition, we have a completely novel set of light responsive cells in the retina called 'intrinsically photoreceptive retinal ganglion cells'. These cells specifically sense changes in light intensity and quality, and have a very important impact on our mood and circadian rhythm.

At this stage, I am unaware of any research that definitively rules out the involvement of these light receptors in our eyes in the activation of melanin in our skin, but given these receptors sense changes in light intensity, perhaps they convey information to the skin cells about how much melanin needs to be released. There are those who believe that our use of sunglasses may actually impact our normal physiological response to sun; there are people who observe that they are less likely to get burned if they are not wearing sunglasses.

Interestingly, in Australia we do so much to reduce our exposure to our harsh sun that as a nation we have developed issues with Vitamin D deficiency. However, what if our 'Slip, Slop, Slap' approach has inadvertently impacted our exposure to light? We absorb light through our eyes and skulls, and we put hats and sunglasses on our babies. We also have 'no hat, no play' policies in our schools, and have had significant campaigns to reduce our risk of skin cancer in Australia for more than 30 years.

What if our need to protect our skin has impacted our mental health?

Obviously, there are a whole bunch of potential reasons for this, and there is ongoing research into many areas of biology and neuroscience. It's incredible the number of new things we are learning all the time; as our technology improves, we are able to learn more about ourselves.

It is really not surprising that when we look to many Indigenous communities around the world, their skin colour is often a good indication of the environmental conditions to which they are native. Melanin is not the only natural protective factor our bodies produce to protect us from the sun, but it does play an important role in the likelihood of developing skin cancers.[30]

Cold therapy

Many of you may have heard of the 'Ice Man' – Wim Hof. He has become an icon in the world of alternative therapies for his use of extreme cold to improve the functioning of his physical body. The things he is able to do, how he reports feeling, and the mental ability he has within himself to survive extremely cold temperatures is nothing short of incredible.

I am not going to pretend to understand everything about what Mr Hof does in his methodology, but suffice to say that he actively encourages the increased use of oxygen in the blood, through controlled breathing techniques and exposure to cold, to assist the body to remain healthy and functioning at its optimum. For many, this method appears to work very effectively for a wide variety of issues – including significant improvements in mental health and the management of pain. The research around his methodology continues to grow.

One of the more interesting elements that has come out of research into his method overturned our scientific understanding of the ability to voluntarily activate the autonomic nervous system and innate immune systems. In particular, the impact on conditions of excessive and persistent inflammation – which results in auto-immune diseases and chronic pain.[31] In other research, the Wim Hof Method has been shown to increase control over key components of the autonomic nervous system, with implications for the benefits of adopted lifestyle interventions that could improve a variety of clinical syndromes.[32]

Electromagnetic stimulation

In varying forms, pulsed electromagnetic fields are used to re-pola-rise cells and assist in reducing inflammation, in turn improving the experience of pain. However, magnetic stimulation is also used to treat severe depression, and the results are quite astonishing.

It makes sense that some change could be reasonably expected from the location of magnetic fields around our body, as the whole Earth is affected by magnetic forces.

Transcranial magnetic stimulation

According to the Mayo Clinic, transcranial magnetic stimulation (TMS) is a non-invasive procedure that uses magnetic fields to stim-ulate nerve cells in the brain to improve symptoms of depression. TMS is typically used when other depression treatments haven't been effective.

During a TMS session, an electromagnetic coil is placed against the scalp near the forehead. The electromagnet painlessly delivers a magnetic pulse that stimulates nerve cells in the region of our brain involved in mood control and depression. It's thought to activate regions of the brain that have decreased activity in depression. TMS is using an energy source to change the way the cells of the brain are functioning.

Though the biology of why TMS works isn't completely under-stood, the stimulation appears to impact how the brain is working, which in turn seems to ease depression symptoms and improve mood. Results for those with long-term mental health issues, often intergenerational depressive conditions, are very positive.

Gut health

There are many supporters of the need for effective gut health to maintain good mental health, and this notion makes sense when we consider that our gut is our 'little brain'. It forms from the same part of the neural tube that our brain develops from, when we are an embryo. We know our gut is clearly involved in common mental health issues because recent research indicates that 95% of our serotonin (the neurotransmitter that is thought to be most involved in feeling good) is developed in our gut.

Recent research supports the fact that diet and gut health affect symptoms expressed by anxiety, stress and depression seen through changes in gut microbiota. As our ability to learn about the functioning of our physical bodies increases, we are learning more about the impact of our psychological expression and our somatic functioning.[33]

We also know that when things are not going well, if we are under extreme stress and we are feeling anxious, our gut can be affected. In most cases, if we have high levels of anxiety, our bowel will become very loose, or bind up tight. It is also common knowledge that when people develop mood disorders, their appetite can be affected — they will either lose weight or gain weight. It is rare that people who are struggling with their mental health would maintain a stable weight.

Food as medicine

There are many and varied examples of being able to improve what ails our bodies by 'fuelling' it correctly. As we are in an obesity epidemic, I don't need to tell you how the reliance on processed foods has impacted our health in the developed world. There is quite a lot of value in considering the way we eat and the impact our food intake has on how we feel within our own bodies.

With the prevalence of 'new' old ways of eating, people are moving away from highly processed foods to eating more protein and less carbohydrates. Most recently there are three popular eating trends that are moving us away from highly processed foods and reinstating the basics:

- *Paleo:* based on the idea we should eat as our ancient hunter-gatherer ancestors did, before we could farm grains or drink milk.

- *Ketogenic:* high protein, high fat and reducing processed carbohydrates.

- *Mediterranean:* clean protein sources with a strong emphasis on fish, wholegrains, good fats and fresh fruit and vegetables.

In recent years, researchers became intrigued by the fact that adults living in regions that border the Mediterranean Sea have the lowest rates of chronic disease and the longest life expectancies in the world.[34] The reasons for this include their diet, but also the fact that they get daily exercise, have a strong connection to family and community, and have a deep appreciation for their quality of life.

Music therapy

Music can be used to regulate mood and arousal in everyday life and to promote physical and psychological health and wellbeing in clinical settings, such as for pain management, relaxation, psychotherapy and personal growth.[35] The notion that 'music is medicine' has roots that extend deep into human history through healing rituals practiced in pre-industrial, tribal-based societies.[36]

Given that music enhances mood and reduces stress, it stands to reason that it may also improve immune function.[37] Claims about the healing power of music are found in many pre-industrial societies and in ancient Greece. The promise of music as therapy is that it is non-invasive, inexpensive, convenient and without side effects.

Music is completely 'natural' and supports links to primal human activities, such as singing. The evidence for the beneficial effects of music on reward, motivation, pleasure, stress, arousal, immunity and social affiliation is mounting.[37]

Music incorporates vibrational tones and facilitates vocal expression — something that humans do from early infancy. It's not just melodic music that shows benefits, we can also benefit from percussive music — such as drumming. Research into drumming circles is growing because they allow for creative self-expression without the need for musical expertise. Participants perform rhythmic sequences of increasing complexity and gradually incorporate directed imagery into their drumming.[35] The physiological impacts from vibration in music can also not be underestimated. Think back to our awareness of emotional vibration, it is not surprising that we respond emotionally to a variety of music sources.

Dance therapy

Dance has been fundamental to human life and culture since the time of our earliest ancestors; a form of self-expression, communication and celebration of life and community.[38] Many cultures utilise dance as a form of expression and community bonding, and it is closely linked to music and vibration, so we can see how dance may be effective in facilitating emotional expression.

In the early-mid 20th century, the formal recognition of dance as a healing modality began. This recognition came with the development of more expressive and improvisational forms of dance popular at that time, as well as the acceptance of the integral relationship between mind and body.

Dance movement therapy emerged as a profession in the US in the 1960s. Dance movement therapy is the relational and therapeutic use of dance and movement to further the physical, emotional, cognitive, social, and cultural functioning of a person.[38]

Ecstatic dance is a form of dance in which the dancers, sometimes without the need to follow specific steps, abandon themselves to the rhythm and move freely as the music takes them, leading to a feeling of ecstasy. Dancers are described as feeling connected to others, and to their own emotional state.[39] The dance serves as a form of meditation, helping people to release tension and manage stress.

EMBODIED SELF-AWARENESS

As more options are developed for integrative approaches in the treatment of our mental health issues, we will see more and more evidence for the interplay between our mind and our bodies.

The key for you to understand about all of these integrative therapies is that we need to be able to build self-awareness about our own challenges and engage in many and varied activities and ways of living that support us to connect to our bodies and our communities, to enable us to feel our best. It is not for anyone else to judge our decisions or tell us 'how' to fix this, nor tell us how we should feel or not feel.

The decision about how we approach our recovery in this life is a combination of many and varied things that help us to feel better – be open, try things out and don't care what anyone else thinks about it!

> *'A sense of spiritual connection allows you*
> *to uplift yourself and everyone around you,*
> *in true self-awareness...*
> *Each expression, each thought, each sentiment*
> *conveys an intuitive wisdom...'*

Kerry Howard, *Define Your Inner Diva*

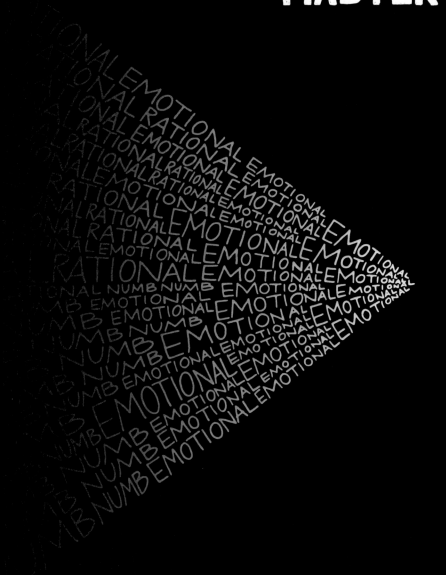

CHAPTER SEVEN
MASTERY

The Impact Of
A Traumatic Experience
Can Be Reduced
If We Process It Early

Throughout this book I have taken you on a journey of understanding how we got into this situation and given you a variety of options to resolve our traumatic experiences and move forward with our lives — in full acceptance of ourselves and others. As you become more self-aware and embodied, you can start to see the familiar patterns and then use these like 'traffic lights' to alert your brain that something has run off the rails.

In chapter three I outlined the basic premise of what I call our 'self-management system'. This is our awareness of our child and protector parts of self, our emerging rational self, and recognising when we have moved into numbing avoidance because we are unable to resolve an issue rationally. This model helps us to manage *any* conflict situation that we get into with another human being.

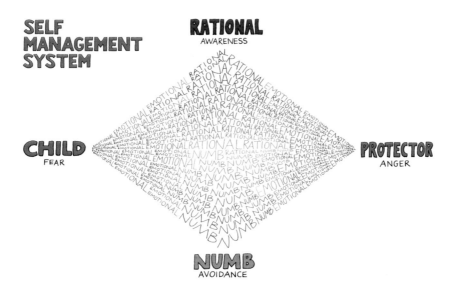

When we have good insight into our own system we are able to cope with any stressor and manage our way through it effectively. That is not to say that we will behave 'perfectly', but we can be aware of our behaviour and be more accepting of our shortcomings as human beings. We are, after all, imperfect!

In better understanding our behaviours and response, we can more readily recognise when situations or circumstances have impacted us or impaired our ability to respond rationally. What I am trying to show everyone is that we are all capable of taking better control over our lives and outcomes but we can't do it unless we learn better self-awareness and learn how to connect with our bodies. Our gut responses are there to protect us – our mind is not only our head, it is our whole upper body, right up through our torso – we just need to learn to listen to it and recognise when we have specific reactions and understand why.

I had a recent situation in which I got to put this process into action – practise what I preach! It was actually in relation to the trip I took to write this book.

I went to Egypt to write; well, at least the majority of it was written there. I also went there when I was writing my first book as I have a good friend who lives there and her beach house is a great space to relax and get the creativity flowing. All was well until I arrived at the airport in Cairo to check in for my return flight.

I had booked through Qantas and everything on my app looked fine. However, when I arrived at Cairo airport at 11 pm for my code-shared return flight to Australia I was told by the Emirates staff that I had no ticket. I won't bore you with the details, but in essence I had changed my return flight with Qantas before I left Australia, but they had not updated my details with Emirates.

In addition, I was also having some staffing issues at home and some other reasons that I needed to return, so when the Emirates staff refused to check me in, I tried to call Qantas and use their short messaging service, but to no avail. I was told that they would not allow me onto the plane – that I needed to call Qantas the following morning. This is when I experienced my first panic attack in more than 20 years!

I began hyperventilating. I developed a dry mouth and my voice changed — I was speaking more rapidly and at a higher pitch. My 'child' was in consciousness... In a complete panic about not being able to get on a flight home when I needed to and feeling lost and afraid about what would happen if I couldn't get home. The only real bonus to this is that the staff got a bit freaked out and called their supervisor over.

The supervisor was trying to assist, but eventually told me that the only way I could get on the flight was if I purchased another ticket — there was only a business class seat and it would be $3500. This is when I disintegrated into panic attack number two! As a result, they assured me that they would find a solution. They gave me some water and tried to find a solution. They offered me a flight with a layover in Dubai; I reaffirmed that I needed to get home on the same flights that I had been booked on.

Eventually, the supervisor instructed me to leave my bags where they were, unattended, and follow him out through security to the ticketing booth, to allow me to pay for my new ticket. I paid for it, including a penalty for purchasing at the airport, and we headed back through security with some level of facilitated access to streamline the process.

As we entered the check-in area, there was a man shouting in Arabic. I wasn't sure what the issue was, but the supervisor rushed to help him and then disappeared out the back... With my passport and my new ticket! I was alone at the check-in counter without a ticket or a passport. My luggage was still sitting on the check-in counter, but there were no staff to check it through — this was 20 minutes before departure! I had to get through immigration and two security check points, through all the duty free shops and who knows how far down the corridor to the plane!

So — I had panic attack number three!

Then a man appeared from the back doors and he asked if he can help me. I explained what I could through my weird breathing and, thankfully, he went to find the supervisor and my passport and new ticket.

Then he told me to follow him. I asked about my bags. He said they would be fine and then there appeared a very young boy, perhaps aged about 10, who dragged my bags down the conveyor. I thought 'I'm never going to see my bags again!' True to his word, he rushed me through more security, immigration, told me what to expect at the next security gate (which didn't happen, so I had to navigate it myself) and sent me on my way.

I was literally running through the duty free shopping area and out to the gate. I was met halfway down the travelator by the Emirates staff member who wouldn't check me in at the counter outside. She said, "Next time, you should check your booking with Qantas before you come to the airport." I was immediately furious, and I pointed out to her that I *did* check my booking. As far as the Qantas app was concerned, everything looked fine.

I decided she was insignificant, but my protector was activated. I finally got to the gate and onto the plane, and as soon as I entered the plane there was a customer service manager who greeted me by asking, "Are you okay Madam?" Well, I immediately burst into tears and commenced panic attack number four! He cleverly got me a bottle of water but he kept the lid (bad idea). They were trying to seat me as they were preparing to push back.

I got to my seat to discover someone else was in it... So, I politely asked if we could please check boarding passes as I thought she was in my allocated seat. She was very gracious about it; apparently someone else had been sitting in her seat and refused to move. She gave up my seat, and when the hostess asked the gentleman at the other end of my aisle to go back to his seat to facilitate this woman having access to the aisle seat that she had already paid for, he refused! He insisted that he would 'pay now' but not move. The hostess walked away at that point.

By this stage, I was out of patience and my protector was out in full force! I just looked at him and in my most direct 'don't mess with me' voice I told him in no uncertain terms that he had to move. In my frustration, the now uncapped bottle of water ended up in my lap. Yet, still he refused to move. When I insisted he just kept complaining, and even told me I was rude! But I wasn't in the mood for his pretentiousness. In the end, he could sense my 'Xena Warrior Princess' was brandishing her broad sword, so he decided to return to his original seat.

The elderly lady wasn't sure which way to look. I apologised to her and told her that if she knew the drama I had been through in the past few hours, she would appreciate why I had lost my patience. She just looked at me and said, "I just wish you had been here half an hour ago. You could have sorted out the man who was sitting in my seat!"

When I arrived in Dubai I discovered that the staff in Cairo had not actually booked me on the same flight and I would have to suffer a 24-hour layover. Bring on panic attack number five! They wouldn't even get me some water when I asked for it. In the end, after another panic attack, I finally got to continue my journey to Australia on my scheduled flight. And they lost my bags, but at least I was on home soil!

Suffice to say that this was the worst travel experience of my life. I hadn't had a panic attack since my bus accident 20 years earlier. However, because I was aware of the issues as I was experiencing them, I haven't had any other panic attacks since.

Some of you may wonder how? Any of you who have ever had a panic attack will know that it's quite a difficult thing to resolve — once the fear is activated in the body, most people feel that they are unable to stop it happening and this often provides a self-fulfilling system where panic attacks become 'normal'. Panic is, after all, just an extreme physical manifestation of fear.

The only reason I was able to manage this experience and leave it behind me as an isolated, yet difficult, experience — was due to the fact that I have very good insight into myself and I understand my parts and how to manage my system. That doesn't mean that I don't have any emotional reactions anymore, but it is very unusual for me to experience strong feelings of shame, fear or anger.

Throughout this experience, my own internal dialogue was assessing everything that was happening and validating my reactions and experiences at every step. I was completely aware that I was feeling overwhelmed and panicked — but inside my head there was a clear conversation going on about how this was completely normal. Literally, I was telling myself that any four year old would be completely freaked out by being stuck in a foreign country in the middle of the night, without any control of the process that would enable me to get to where I needed to be — on that plane!

I know my system and I had a good map to understand what was happening and why. As a result, all of the thinking dialogue that was going in my head after I got on the plane was validating — it didn't leave me with any sort of traumatic injury.

Intervening early

Research shows that our brains start to consolidate information within the first six hours after a traumatic event, so one of the first steps in self-awareness is the ability to undertake some activities that can help to minimise the impact of our experiences.

When we get stressed, we often talk things over with someone close to us. We are looking for engagement with others and support for our experience, seeking a connection that validates our perspective. We are reacting to the impact of an external stressor on our system and we are seeking a supportive connection to ensure our perspective is supported. In short, the stressor creates the potential for a disconnection, and the connection with our friends and family through telling them the story is designed to facilitate our processing of the problem as we either get confirmation of how the experience was unreasonable and the problem is external, or we get confirmation that we did something wrong and the issue is internal.

Our usual approach is to get a friend on the phone or go home and speak with our partner. What is important to understand is that storytelling activates emotion. This emotional activation is important for processing the impact of the stressor. In my case, I ended up speaking to the lady who was now seated next to me about my ordeal to that point. She empathised with my experience, which helped me feel justified in my approach. In talking through it I could feel the panic starting to leave my body, but it wasn't enough to just talk it through — in order to best facilitate processing, we need to engage in bilateral stimulation.

Bilateral stimulation

Bilateral stimulation is the basis of EMDR Therapy, but it can be facilitated in a number of ways. In essence, we need to get our body stimulated in a side-to-side movement or activation. In EMDR Therapy we use eye movement, auditory music or tones that go from one ear to the other, or physical stimulation of the hands or arms.

So, when I was on the plane and I had told my story but I could still feel the tension in my body, I decided that I needed to get up and move my body. I made the conscious decision to go down the back of the plane and try to walk around a bit, but I knew that I needed to think about the experience while I was moving. So, I started thinking over the whole experience again, like a video in my head, moving my feet and hands down the side of my legs, first one side then the other. It didn't take very long for me to feel a sense of calm. I felt completely justified in my behaviour throughout the experience.

When I arrived in Dubai I was very calm. When I had the second issue of the flight mix-up, I walked around the duty free area of the airport going over the situation on the phone with my partner and then sat down and recorded a Facebook live post about my experience. I was able to gain validity of my experience, and in walking around while I told my story I was able to reduce my arousal. I felt completely accepting of my emotional responses, so there wasn't any issue that needed to keep my arousal high.

RAW

The impact of a stressful or traumatic experience can be reduced if we get onto it early. There are some simple things that we can do for ourselves to help reduce the impact of these events. I have created a simple mnemonic to remind us how to work through our traumatic experiences as they occur in our life: RAW.

Reality

It is important to obtain a reality check about the situation as early as we possibly can. This is why we reach out to friends and family when things happen to us. We need to make sure that our behaviour was appropriate and justified — we need validation.

Even if we have done something wrong, we can talk through the 'why' we behaved in an unexpected way, and through this process we learn to understand ourselves and accept our little idiosyncrasies. This is important for us as individuals, but it is very important in community trauma.

When we experience community-wide traumatic events, we will often compare our situation to that of another and find ourselves feeling better, or worse, but it doesn't feel as personal. This is an important step in trying to process this type of trauma because the situation is difficult, but I am not the only one involved or affected, so the impact is mediated.

Awareness

We need to be aware of our own behaviour. It seems obvious, but when we first start to build awareness, we have to understand that we have natural defence mechanisms that don't like to feel responsible for negative situations.

To assist this process, we need to pay attention to our language and behaviour. Is our voice high pitched and fast? Are we being quiet and not saying anything? Either extreme indicates that we are highly aroused – if talking loudly and emotionally then our protector is activated, seeking validation for the unfairness. If quiet, we're likely in child mode, overwhelmed or feeling responsible for the situation. The only other observation here might be quiet anger – this is usually when we're unable to obtain validation from an external source and we stop trying to justify our position because we feel like there is no point.

Walk 'n' talk

At the very minimum, it is important to talk it over with a friend while walking. Walking facilitates bilateral stimulation and processing. Bilateral stimulation is scientifically proven to reduce the impact of traumatic experiences.

I'm sure you are aware that if you get into an argument with your partner, you'll go and talk to a friend about what they did – seeking validation. Rather than doing this over a coffee, try going for a walk instead – in this way you will be able to work through the issues with your partner's behaviour, rather than having coffee with six different friends, repeating the same story, but not able to work through it.

Self-management system

I have turned the self-management system illustration into a hand-out for clients, you can obtain a copy for yourself as part of the resources that I outline in the 'Next Steps' at the end of this book. Designed to be printed in colour and laminated, you can then put it on the fridge, on your bedside table or behind the toilet door – somewhere where you can be reminded to 'check in' whenever you find yourself triggered and expressing frustration or feeling like you want to stay in bed and pull the doona over your head!

This diagram operates like a map – when we notice that we're emotional, for any reason, we can use this as an opportunity to identify where in this system we are and then we need to work out how to get ourself moving towards 'rational'.

Whenever we find ourselves in conflict with another human being – our partner, family member or colleague – we are able to utilise the awareness of our self-management system to establish more awareness about what's going on.

When we experience strong emotion it can be very easy to just get caught up in the moment and use our re-telling of the story to keep seeking validation from external sources, but ultimately if we want to be able to resolve the situation we need to be able to manage it for ourselves. We need to make it an internal examination of what is going on.

Are we sad and crying (child) or are we frustrated and raising our voice (protector) – by simply reflecting on our behaviour we can start to see where we sit in this map. With awareness we are then able to take action to move ourself more towards the rational, where our thinking is clear and calm and we are making plans to resolve the issue and move forward. It's important to remember that we can only move forward if the person we are in conflict with is also willing to move forward with us. If not, we will find ourself moving into numbing to avoid the decision to take a different path to the other person.

This happens a lot in our interpersonal relationships with partners. There is usually a 'common' trigger point that sends us into child or protector mode. Recall that we can move between these emotional responses, even vacillate from frustration to crying, and back again, before we are able to calm yourself and move towards rational. However, we can only move towards rational *if* our partner is also prepared to move into rational with us – that they agree on how we can resolve this and they are willing to take action along with us. If they don't agree on the action needed, or they need time to demonstrate proof of their action, then we need to move into numbing to cope with the situation now.

It's really important here to focus on the fact that this is *your* self-management system – the person we are having difficulties with has their own system and they need to manage it themselves. However, once we understand this system it makes it really easy to see how conflicts arise and how to mitigate them more effectively.

MASTERING THE SYSTEM

The reality of any situation is that self-aware people are constantly trying to move themselves forward; they want to grow and embody rational awareness. There are many people in the world who prefer to externalise everything; they don't grow or change because they operate in constant numbing – avoiding responsibility and stagnating their life. We all know people like this and they're not the ones reading this book! These people can't acknowledge that their problems might actually rest with them – it's easier to blame everyone else.

When we understand the system and how conflicts arise, we can approach each situation with curious observation about our own behaviour. Like when I was in the airport having a panic attack,

I recall observing my hyperventilation and tears as identifying markers that my child mode was activated. I was then able to talk to myself as any caring adult would a frightened child, with care and concern and reassurance that the adult in me could work this out and I didn't need to worry. In this way I was able to calm myself down, rather than buying into the fear and having it escalate — or worse, berating myself for being a pathetic cry–baby. In this way, I was able to settle my emotions much faster.

It will take a while for this level of self–awareness to grow in us and we may need to engage in some therapy along the way to help ourself along. However, the key to getting the most from this is in reinforcing the awareness of our place in each conflict situation — even if it is 'after' the fact. That is why I say to refer to this as a map. When we first start to put this reflective process in place it will be after we have had an argument with our partner or parent, or experienced conflict at work. Rather than berating ourself, try to put our rational hat on and see if we can understand the process we went through — not just for our behaviour but also for the other person.

As we become more familiar with the patterns of emotional activation, we can begin to see how 'both' people in a conflict situation are operating from one of these four modes, and they may jump between them over the course of any discussion.

When clients enter therapy, I outline to them that the 'emotional' areas in the map are usually where they are spending the majority of their time; that's why they seek to engage in therapy — they want help to 'stop feeling' so strongly, all the time. The challenge is that most people are looking for the solution to eliminate the feelings, repress them and make them go away, as this is how we have been taught to manage our emotions all of our lives.

I hope what I have been able to show you is that this approach doesn't work and is fraught with difficulty — for our health and happiness. We need to understand our emotional responses, validate our experiences and rationally move things forward. However, we need to recognise that we can only move forward *if* the other person moves forward with us, or we take an action that means that our desired outcome is no longer dependent on that person to provide.

With a partner this may mean that we separate, or in work we may choose to find another job. These two examples are indicative of spending too much time in numbing avoidance and realising that the other person is never going to embrace change and work with us rationally to enable us to get what we want. When the 'other' isn't coming to the party, we either have to make the decision to change what it is that we want, or seek to obtain it elsewhere.

For many people, constantly moving from one situation to another is how they have managed to avoid rational awareness and the need to change their behaviour. These are often the externalisers – constantly blaming others for their issues and never taking the time to work through their interpersonal challenges. It usually takes something significant to happen in their lives to alter this pattern of behaviour.

The opposing position is to constantly internalise responsibility for every conflict, blaming ourself for the behaviour of everyone around us – as we see ourself as the source of all of the issues that our family and friends have. These extremes are just as destructive as each other – we need balance.

Conflict situations provide us an opportunity to learn, gain insight into ourselves and others and work rationally to clearly identify what is our responsibility and what is the responsibility of others. As we embrace this journey, we will help others to understand themselves along the way because we will start to handle conflict in very different ways. By taking responsibility for ourself, we are able to more effectively communicate our needs and desires, but we are also aware that the responsibility for having them met is ours. If they can't be met by one person, they may be met by another.

I don't mean we should abandon all relationships — on the contrary. Recall at the very beginning of this book I outlined that we need connections to sustain life and it is our traumatic experiences that create disconnection. Now that we are more aware of how our traumatic experiences have impacted our life, it affords us the opportunity to notice their impact on our ability to have our needs met. If my partner is unable to meet a particular need, perhaps I can get this need met by a friend or family member. Alternatively, I might engage in some therapy to try to understand the need, potentially to resolve it.

Ultimately, we need to be aware that we have to take responsibility for addressing these needs, understanding what drives them and working towards a rational solution for resolving them.

'I am the master of my fate,
I am the captain of my soul.'

William Ernest Henley

NEXT STEPS

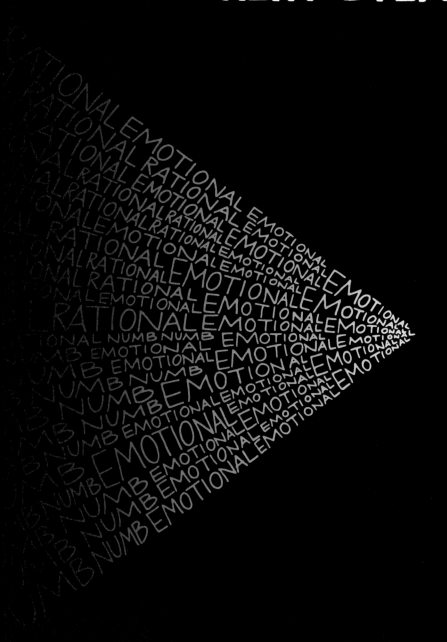

We need a purpose for our recovery!
I want to help you find that purpose

I hope that in reading this book you have been able to understand why trauma is at the basis of all of our psychological and physiological issues. When we take action and engage in a number of different therapeutic processes we learn to be fully embodied and develop more self-awareness.

Throughout this book I have outlined how we got to be here and given us some ideas about the kinds of activities that we can engage with to manage our own mental health and wellbeing. However, none of this information will make any difference unless we make a plan to change our approach.

THE POWER OF THREE

You will recall in chapter six I outlined the power of three in making change. My challenge to you is to set some goals that you are wanting to achieve in the next three weeks, six weeks, three months and six months — significant markers that will assist you to increase your sense of connection, improve your self-awareness and begin to feel empowered to develop mastery over your life.

I outlined in chapter two about how the nodes of the central nervous system, the chakras and meridians overlap. When you look at the updated diagram on the next page, I hope you can now see how the chapters in this book have been structured to assist you to build awareness about your body systems and how you can enhance your management of this system.

BODY SYSTEMS OVERLAP

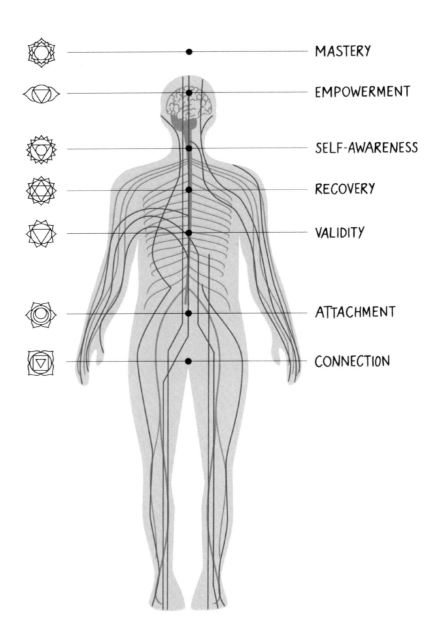

MASTERY

EMPOWERMENT

SELF-AWARENESS

RECOVERY

VALIDITY

ATTACHMENT

CONNECTION

Who, what, when, where, why and how!

I want to support you to take action, to move forward in your journey to achieving mastery over your system. Research[40] shows that merely setting a goal is not enough. Your chances of success in achieving your goals are mediated by a number of factors. The probability of success increases with accountability, as follows:

- 10% — If you have an actual idea or goal — the 'what'

- 25% — If you consciously decide you will do it — the 'where'

- 40% — If you decide when you will do it — the 'when'

- 50% — If you plan how you will do it — the 'how'

- 65% — If you commit to someone, you will do it — the 'who'

- 95% — If you have a specific accountability appointment with a person you've committed to — the 'why'

Find your 'Why'…

You should get onto the website — www.thetroublewithtrauma.com and on the 'Next Steps' page you will find the resources to help you take action and recover.

BETTER BUSINESS, BETTER LIFE, BETTER WORLD

WRITTEN BY
KERRY HOWARD, DANIEL PRIESTLEY, MASAMI SATO, PAUL DUNN
AND OTHER INSPIRING BUSINESS LEADERS

Better business
Better life
Better world

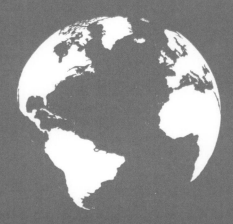

EDITED BY
JONATHAN PIPE, KATIE PIPE AND LAURA PIPE

Understand yourself and embrace difference

Based in Australia, Kerry Howard AKA Ms Pink Herself is:

- A psychologist, executive coach, entrepreneur, mother, daughter and luminary. She has worked with 500+ clients to improve their sense of self and find their joy in life
- Releasing her first book at the end of 2016 – the culmination of her life's work in the Personal Transformation space
- Absolutely passionate about helping people to experience their best life, even when they are not sure it is possible
- A charismatic keynote presenter. She draws on her own life experiences and practice to deliver powerful messages in a truly authentic way - presenting on a diverse range of topics including women in business, personal growth, relationships, health and wellbeing, trauma, career transition and life transformation

Here is the advice she would give to her grandchildren...

Better business

Follow your passion!

Make a business out of the thing you love most, or are most interested in, as it is really very difficult to commit yourself to the demands of running a business if you do not enjoy what you are doing every day.

Finding your passion can be quite a difficult thing to do, though, especially when you are young. It is also important to understand that over our lifetime our interests, and therefore our passions, will change... so don't be afraid to move on from your business when the passion for it starts to wane and you find yourself with a new interest.

You are a creative and inspiring individual and your business, when based on your passion, will always reflect that creativity. As a result, your passion and creativity will allow you to inspire those around you.

111

Better life

Love does NOT conquer all!

We are raised to believe that we have a soul mate in the world somewhere and we are destined to find him or her and live happily ever after...

Perhaps there is, and perhaps you will.

But if you really want to know how to achieve long-term success in an intimate relationship, you have to recognise that love does not conquer all things - we really need to check if we share values, beliefs, behaviours and attitudes to ensure the success of our relationships.

Even when you are young, if you believe that one day you might like to marry or make a long term commitment to the person that you are dating, it is essential that you spend some time exploring some of the 'key' areas of married life before you contemplate formalising that commitment.

You need to understand your partner's values, about money, assets, leisure time, children and their education, working life and career progression, travel and ideals of home life. Along with where you want to live, how you expect to live there and the obligations that all of these decisions place on you as the individuals within your relationship.

You need to know your love languages and know how to show the other one that you love them in 'their' love languages, and they commit to reciprocating.

A long-term intimate relationship is like a business partnership with sex thrown in. You would never go into a business relationship with someone without understanding their vision and plans for the future of the business, their aspirations, their time commitment to the business and their financial contribution and how this compares with your own vision. You compare this with your own contribution and determine the percentage of ownership of the business accordingly.

An intimate relationship also requires this level of analysis to ensure it is successful. This is not 'un-romantic' or overly analytical. It is simply an insightful way to ensure the long-term success of your union, and provides a loving and stable environment for the next generation.

Love enhances all of our values, attitudes, beliefs and behaviours... which is why we need to ensure a shared understanding of what ours are, and if they are compatible with the person you love.

112

REFERENCES

1. Schacter, D L, Gilbert, D T and Wegner, D M. (2011). *Psychology*. New York: Worth. 2nd Edition.

2. Maslow, A H. (1968). *Toward a Psychology of Being*. New York: D. Van Nostrand Company.

3. Daniels, M. (1982). *The development of the concept of self-actualization in the writings of Abraham Maslow*. Springer-Verlag, Current Psychological Reviews, Vol. 2, pp. 61–75.

4. Maslow, A H. (1943). *A Theory of Human Motivation*. Psychological Review, 50(4), 370–396. https://doi.org/10.1037/h0054346

5. Brown, B. (2012). *Daring Greatly: How the Courage to Be Vulnerable Transforms the Way We Live, Love, Parent, and Lead*. New York: Gotham Books.

6. Nadler, S. (2015). *The Philosopher, the Priest, and the Painter: A Portrait of Descartes*. New Jersey: Princeton University Press.

7. Cunning, D. (2014). *The Cambridge Companion to Descartes' Meditations*. Cambridge: Cambridge University Press, 2014.

8. Pert, C. (1999). *Molecules Of Emotion: The Science Behind Mind-Body Medicine*. New York: Touchstone.

9. Fogel, A. (2013). *Body Sense: The Science and Practice of Embodied Self-Awareness*. New York: W W Norton & Company.

10. Lovelock, J E. (1979). *Gaia, a new look at life on earth*. New York: Oxford University Press.

11. United Nations. *The Global Goals For Sustainable Development*. The Global Goals. [Online] United Nations. [Cited: 27 July 2019.] https://www.globalgoals.org/.

12. Rotter, J B. (1966). *Generalized expectancies for internal versus external control of reinforcement.* American Psychological Association, Psychological Monographs: General and Applied, Vol. 80, pp. 1–28.

13. Carlson, N R, Buskist, W, Heth, C D, and Schmaltz, R. (2009). Psychology: *The Science of Behaviour.* Pearson Education Canada. Fourth Canadian Edition.

14. Kirk, P J D. (2016). *Quantum Lite Simplified: How to calm the chaos.* The Magic of Quantum.

15. Melzack, R and Wall, P D. (1965). *Pain Mechanisms: A New Theory.* Science, Vol. 150, pp. 971–979. DOI: 10.1126/science.150.3699.971.

16. Johnsen, T J and Friborg, O. (2015). *The Effects of Cognitive Behavioral Therapy as an Anti-Depressive Treatment is Falling: A Meta-Analysis.* Psychological Bulletin, Vol. 141, pp. 747–768.

17. Michie, S. (2005). *Is Cognitive Behaviour Therapy Effective for Changing Health Behaviours? Commentary on Hobbis and Sutton.* London : Sage Publications, Journal of Health Psychology, Vol. 10, pp. 33–36.

18. Holmes, J. (2002). *All you need is cognitive behaviour therapy?* BMJ, Vol. 324, pp. 288–294.

19. Shapiro, F. (2014). *The Role of Eye Movement Desensitization and Reprocessing (EMDR) Therapy in Medicine: Addressing the Psychological and Physical Symptoms Stemming from Adverse Life Experiences.* The Permanente Journal, Vol. 18, pp. 71–77.

20. Lipton, B H. (2016). *The biology of belief: unleashing the power of consciousness, matter & miracles.* Carlsbad, California: Hay House Inc.

21. Boeree, C G. (2018). *Personality Theories: From Freud to Frankl.* CreateSpace Independent Publishing Platform.

22. The Buddhist Centre. [Online] [Cited: 10 January 2020.] https://thebuddhistcentre.com/text/what-meditation.

23. Wang, Y T, Huang, G, Duke, G and Yang, Y. (2017). *Tai Chi, Yoga, and Qigong as Mind–Body Exercises*. Evidence–Based Complementary and Alternative Medicine, Article ID 8763915. https://doi.org/10.1155/2017/8763915

24. Young, J S, Cashwell, C S and Giordano, A L. (2010). *Breathwork as a Therapeutic Modality: An Overview for Counselors*. Counseling and Values, Vol. 55, pp. 113–125.

25. Cohen, K S. (2000) *The Way of QiGong*. New York: Random House.

26. Dayanidhi, Y S G and Dayanidhi, S R. (2002). *Principles and Methods of Yoga Practices*. [ed.] Dr Ananda Balayogi Bhavanani. Puducherry, India: International Centre for Yoga Education and Research.

27. Satyananda Yoga Academy (2011) *Vision Australasia*. Satyananda Yoga Academy.

28. Asher, G N, Gerkin, J and Gaynes, B N. (2017). *Complementary Therapies for Mental Health Disorders*. Medical Clinics, Vol. 101, pp. 847–864.

29. Jurvelin, H. (2018). *Transcranial Bright Light – The Effect on Human Psychophysiology*. Doctoral dissertation D 1450, University of Oulu. Repository. http://jultika.oulu.fi/files/isbn9789526218113.pdf [Online] [Cited: https://humancharger.com/research/].

30. Brenner, M and Hearing, V J. (2008). *The Protective Role of Melanin Against UV Damage in Human Skin*. Photochemistry and photobiology, Vol. 84, pp. 539–549.

31. Kox, M, van Eijk, L T, Zwaag, J, van den Wildenberg, J, Sweep, F C, van der Hoeven, J G and Pickkers, P. (2014). *Voluntary activation of the sympathetic nervous system and attenuation of the innate immune response in humans*. Proceedings of the National Academy of Sciences of the United States of America, Vol. 111, pp. 7379–84. doi: 10.1073/pnas.1322174111.

32. Muzik, O, Reilly, K T and Diwadkar, V A. (2018). *Brain over body – a study on the willful regulation of autonomic fuction during cold exposure*. NeuroImage, Vol. 172, pp. 632–641.

33. Schnorr, S L and Bachner, H A. (2016). *Integrative Therapies in Anxiety Treatment with Special Emphasis on the Gut Microbiome.* Yale Journal of Biology and Medicine, Vol. 89, pp. 397–422.

34. Martinez–Gonzalez, M A and Martin–Calvo, N. (2016). *Mediterranean diet and life expectancy; beyond olive oil, fruits and vegetables.* Current Opinion in clinical Nutrition and Metabolic Care, Vol. 19, pp. 401–407.

35. Chanda, M L and Levitin, D J. (2013). *The Neurochemistry of Music.* Cell Press, Trends in Cognitive Sciences, Vol. 17, pp. 180–194.

36. Merriam, A P. (1964). *The Anthropology of Music.* Nortthwestern University Press. ISBN 0-8101-0607-8.

37. Koelsch, S and Stegemann, T. (2012). *The brain and positive biological effects in healthy and clinical populations.* [book auth.] MacDonald, R A R, Kreutz, G and Mitchell, L. Music, health and wellbeing. Oxford University Press.

38. Dance Movement Therapy Association of Australasia. *Dance Movement Therapy.* [Online] [Cited: 14 June 2020.] https://dtaa.org. au/therapy/.

39. Zmolek, P and Zmolek, J A. (2002). Dance as Ecstatic Ritual/Theatre. Callous Physical Theatre. [Cited: 14 June 2020.] http:// callousphysicaltheatre.weebly.com/uploads/1/6/1/5/16155000/ destatic.pdf.

40. Phillips, P P. (2010) *ASTD Handbook for Measuring and Evaluating Training.* American Society for Training & Development.

ABOUT KERRY HOWARD

Kerry Howard is a best-selling author, psychologist and trauma prevention strategist. She developed *The Trouble with Trauma* as the culmination of her life's work in helping people to understand that trauma is a normal part of our lives as human beings. That we just need to understand it's impact and implement processes to improve our awareness and allow us to resolve our challenges.

Kerry is also a divorcee and single mother of two daughters, a sister and a daughter – she developed the humorous *Why Men Are Like Shoes* as an analogy to explain the concept of dating to her youngest daughter when Kerry started dating again, following her divorce.

It is an irreverent look at dating for women, using an analogy that most women understand – a love of 'shoes'. Kerry is passionate about helping people to experience their best life, even when they are not sure it is possible, and that includes having fun with dating and relationships.

Kerry is a psychologist, executive coach and a self-confessed 'definitive diva'. In her private practice, Kerry has worked with 1000+ clients to improve their sense of self and find their joy in life and improve their relationships.

Kerry is also a charismatic keynote presenter. She draws on her own life experiences and practice to deliver powerful messages in a truly authentic way. Kerry presents on a diverse range of topics including mental health, personal growth and life transformation.

Kerry has an absolute love of being able to assist people to turn their lives around.

"I get pure joy from being able to give somebody a different perspective of themselves and see them make significant change and truly believe it. It's wonderful to see that light bulb moment in their eyes, when they finally understand why they've been doing the same thing over and over and over again and why they don't have to do it anymore! It's awesome when an individual can start seeing themselves in a completely different way, really like who they are, and change their lives as a result."

Put simply, Kerry provides profoundly simple, yet often humorous insights that are changing the way thousands of people think about their mental health and their lives.

For more background information please visit **kerryannhoward. com/books**

Also by Kerry Howard

Define Your Inner Diva meets the growing demand for simple, practical and effective advice for professional, single women to better understand themselves and clearly define what they seek in life, as well as providing guidance on how to be healthy, find successful and supportive relationships and live luscious lives.

The value of understanding ourselves is not always clear in relation to how we treat ourselves, how we interact with others, or how we find our best balance in order to feel that life is fun, enriching and fulfilling.

This book resolves the issues that currently exist within the self-help industry, which focuses on individual problems and doesn't provide a comprehensive review and exploration process by which successful women can understand why they have been able to achieve career satisfaction, but not achieve optimal health, full meaning in life, or find their most supportive life partners.

Kerry's approach in this book is unique due to its semi-autobiographical nature; it is peppered with her experiences in applying this information to her own life. Kerry has made this journey herself and assisted over 1000+ others to do so as well. This book comes from a place of practical experience and credibility across all forms of personal transformation.

Kerry provides down-to-earth advice for professional women on every aspect of the life review process from self, relationships, career, finances, health and wellbeing and spirit. *Define Your Inner Diva* is the answer for those women who have always wanted to be truly happy, focused on their health and satisfied in their bodies, who seek to gain a supportive partner who loves and respects their unique value and contribution to the world.

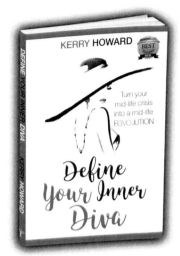

Also by Kerry Howard

The dating scene is fraught with difficulty for all the single ladies.

Why Men Are Like Shoes is an irreverent and fun book, it takes a humorous look at men and compares them to shoes. This book is designed for all of the gorgeous single girls to compare something that they know and love – Shoes, to something they love, but often don't understand so well – Men!

Alternatively, she may appreciate an understanding of why she is unable to 'settle' for only one pair of shoes – when it is obvious that her wardrobe requires 'multiple' pairs.

This book takes a 'tongue in cheek' look at why some woman NEED many pairs of shoes, and what a girl needs to consider if she is wanting to find her 'perfect' pair.

The perfect gift for your girlfriend, sister, daughter or mother – this book helps to explain why she may not have found her perfect guy yet, but gives her some pointers on what she needs to be looking for in order to allow her to find him, or to confirm why she doesn't need to settle for only one pair.

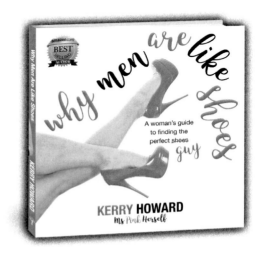